Invariant Measurement with Explanatory Rasch Models in the Human Sciences

George Engelhard · Stefanie A. Wind

Invariant Measurement with Explanatory Rasch Models in the Human Sciences

Springer

George Engelhard
University of Georgia
Athens, GA, USA

Stefanie A. Wind
University of Alabama
Tuscaloosa, AL, USA

ISBN 978-3-032-08815-4 ISBN 978-3-032-08816-1 (eBook)
https://doi.org/10.1007/978-3-032-08816-1

This Springer imprint is published by the registered company Springer Nature Switzerland AG
The registered company address is: Gewerbestrasse 11, 6330 Cham, Switzerland

To my family: Judy Monsaas, Emily Monsaas Engelhard, David Monsaas Engelhard, Shimby McCreery, Dashiell Engelhard McCreery, and Cassio Engelhard McCreery. My love for you is invariant! (George Engelhard, Jr.)

To Fred. I love you more than I can explain! (Stefanie A. Wind)

Preface

Stevens (1951) once stated that the "scientist seeks measures that will stay put while his back is turned" (p. 21). This search for the discovery or creation of scales in the human sciences that meets this condition is one of the most difficult aspects of research in the human sciences. How do we measure school achievement, social attitudes, and other keys aspects of human behavior in a meaningful and useful way? Although there are a variety of perspectives on measurement in the human sciences, Rasch measurement theory provides a framework for developing scales that have the potential to meet the requirements of invariant measurement. Rasch stated these conditions as follows:

> The comparison between two stimuli should be independent of which particular individuals were instrumental for the comparison; and it should also be independent of which stimuli within the considered class were or might also have been compared.
>
> Symmetrically, a comparison between two individuals should be independent of which particular stimuli with the class considered were instrumental for the comparison; and it should also be independent of which other individuals were also compared on the same or on some other occasion (Rasch, 1961, pp. 331–332)

These two requirements reflect person-invariant item calibration and item-invariant person measurement. The basic idea is that under appropriate conditions, items can be located on a line representing a latent variable that is conditionally independent of the persons used to collect the item response data. Symmetrically, it follows that persons can be located on the same line in a way that is independent of the particular items. Each of these ideas will be described in more detail within this book.

The search for invariant measures also includes a specification of the conditions under which invariance is not obtained. Simply fitting Rasch models does not guarantee invariance without systematic study of these conditions. In this book, Rasch measurement theory is described with an eye toward discovering the conditions where our measures are invariant, and if not, then identifying the variables that may limit this invariance. There have been exciting new developments based on extensions of Rasch measurement theory that include item and person covariates. These various extensions of Rasch models can provide for a framework for consideration of invariant relationships. To paraphrase Stevens (1951), scientists seek *relationships between measures* that stay put when their backs are turned.

Overview of Chapters

An overview of the chapters in this book is shown in Fig. 1. This figure reflects the basic structure of this book. Chapter 1 introduces the general themes of this book. This includes a discussion of Rasch measurement theory, and an illustrative analysis using the Dichotomous Model to the analyze a scale for measuring learning stimulation in home environments.

Chapters 2 and 3 present the basic foundations of Rasch measurement theory. Specifically, Chapter 2 develops the historical and philosophical principles of Rasch measurement theory. This chapter includes a discussion of invariant measurement, and the basic principles underlying the family of Rasch models. The implications of these Rasch principles related to measurement, explanation, and invariance are considered throughout the book.

Chapter 3 focuses on the estimation of the Dichotomous Model using generalized linear mixed models. A brief summary is provided of linear models, mixed models, generalized linear models, and generalized linear mixed models. The underlying statistical framework of generalized linear mixed models is presented for estimating the parameters of the Dichotomous Model.

Evaluation of measurement quality is based on model-data fit, and this issue is addressed in Chap. 4. It is essential to evaluate measurement quality based on model-data fit. Model-data fit is organized around various statistical and graphical analyses of residuals. It is important to recognize that the invariance properties of Rasch measurement theory are only achieved when good model-data fit is obtained.

The use of generalized linear mixed models for estimating explanatory Rasch models is introduced in Chap. 5. This chapter provides specific details about linear logistic Rasch models and latent regression Rasch models. This chapter also describes in detail the descriptive and explanatory versions of these models.

Chapter 6 addresses both descriptive and explanatory Rasch measurement theory within the context of rater-mediated assessments. Chapter 7 describes the steps that can be used when a researcher is constructing a scale based on the principles of Rasch measurement theory. Next, Chap. 8 provides a compact introduction to rating scale analysis for polytomous explanatory Rasch models.

Finally, the conclusion summarizes the main ideas of the book, and provides suggestions for future research and practice for next generation measurement in the human sciences.

Athens, GA, USA George Engelhard
Tuscaloosa, AL, USA Stefanie A. Wind

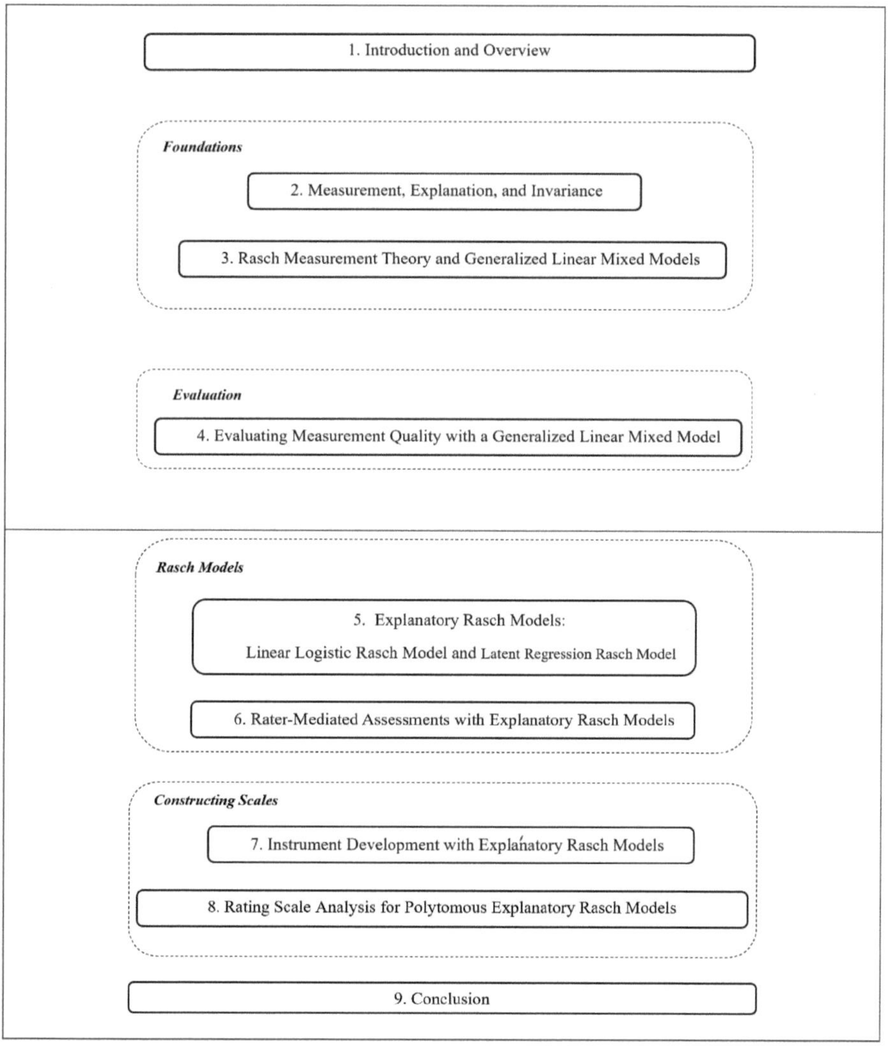

Fig. 1 Overview of the chapters

References

Rasch, G. (1961). On general laws and meaning of measurement in psychology. In J. Neyman (Ed.), *Proceedings of the fourth Berkeley Symposium on mathematical statistics and probability* (pp. 321-333). University of California Press.

Stevens, S. S. (1951). Mathematics, measurement and psychophysics. In S. S. Stevens (Ed.), *Handbook of experimental psychology* (pp. 1-49). Wiley.

Competing Interests The authors have no competing interests to declare that are relevant to the content of this manuscript.

Contents

1 **Introduction** 1

2 **Measurement, Explanation, and Invariance** 15

3 **Rasch Measurement Theory and Generalized Linear Mixed Models** 49

4 **Evaluating Measurement Quality for Dichotomous Rasch Models** 63

5 **Explanatory Rasch Models: Linear Logistic Rasch Models and Latent Regression Rasch Models** 93

6 **Rater-Mediated Assessments with Explanatory Rasch Models** 113

7 **Instrument Development with Explanatory Rasch Models** 157

8 **Rating Scale Analysis for Polytomous Explanatory Rasch Models** 187

9 **Conclusion** 213

Index 219

About the Authors

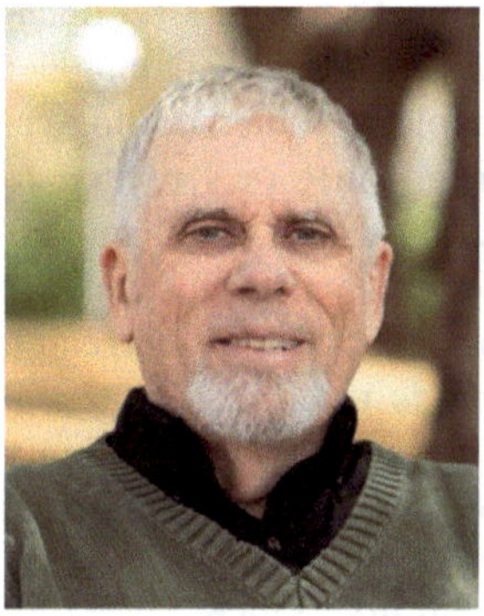

Professor George Engelhard, Jr., Ph.D joined the faculty at The University of Georgia in the fall of 2013. He is professor emeritus at Emory University (1985 to 2013). Professor Engelhard received his Ph.D. in 1985 from The University of Chicago (MESA Program—measurement, evaluation, and statistical analysis). While at the University of Chicago, he worked with Professors Ben Bloom and Ben Wright. His research has focused on a variety of topics including invariant measurement; the role of assessment in improving educational processes; Rasch measurement theory; rater-mediated assessments; history of measurement theory; assessment of written composition; and measurement of food insecurity (nationally and internationally). Professor Engelhard has published three books. He is the co-editor of four edited books, and author or co-author of over 200 journal articles, book chapters, and monographs. He serves on several national technical advisory committees on educational measurement and policy including Georgia and New Jersey. He has served as President of the Georgia Educational Research Association (1992–93). He has received several awards and fellowships including a National Academy of Education/Spencer Foundation Fellowship Award, a Lilly Post-Doctoral Teaching Award, and Sears Writing across the Curriculum Project Award. In 2015, he received the first Qiyas Award for Excellence in International Educational Assessment recognizing his contributions to the field of education based on his book (*Invariant measurement: Using Rasch models in the social, behavioral, and health sciences*), as well as his program of research that focuses on the improvement of educational measurement at the local, national, and international levels. He was the 2018 recipient of Benjamin Drake Wright Senior Scholar Award from the American Educational Research Association. He is an elected fellow of the American Educational Research Association. He is a past president of the Pacific Rim Objective Measurement Society (PROMS). He recently published with Jue Wang a book entitled: *Rasch models for solving measurement problems: Invariant measurement in the social sciences.*

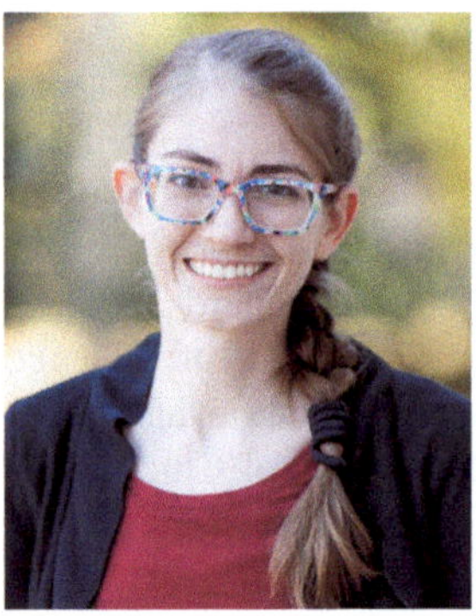

Professor Stefanie A. Wind, Ph.D., received her Ph.D. in Educational Measurement from Emory University in 2014. She is currently a Professor of Educational Measurement at the University of Alabama. Her primary research involves exploring methodological issues in measurement, focusing on topics related to rater-mediated assessments, rating scales, Rasch models and item response theory models, and nonparametric item response theory. She also conducts applied research in which she uses these methods to address practical questions and challenges in a variety of disciplinary areas related to education. Professor Wind has published four books and over 150 peer-reviewed journal articles, along with chapters in edited volumes. She has received several awards for her research, including the Alicia Cascallar Award from the National Council on Measurement in Education, and the Georg William Rasch Early Career Publication Award from the Rasch Measurement Special Interest Group of the American Educational Research Association. She has also received awards for teaching in educational measurement, including the Nellie Rose McCrory Faculty Excellence Award in Teaching and the Innovative Teaching Award from the University of Alabama. She currently serves in several editorial roles, including as Associate Editor for *Measurement and Evaluation in Counseling and Development*, and Editor of *Teaching Educational Research Methods*, and serves on the editorial boards for several other journals. She is currently serving as Chair of the Rasch Measurement Special Interest Group of the American Educational Research Association, and program co-chair for the 2026 meeting of the National Council on Measurement in Education.

List of Figures

Fig. 1.1 Generic variable map. *Note* Categories indicate subgroups of persons (e.g., male/female), while classifications indicate subsets of items (e.g., adult-/child-dominated activities) 6
Fig. 1.2 Three item response functions (IRFs) for Guttman and Rasch Scales with three persons (θ = -2, 0, 2) 7
Fig. 1.3 Variable map for learning stimulation scale. *Note* Home data (40 homes, 11 items, focus of activities: A = adult-dominated activities, and C = child-dominated activities) 10
Fig. 2.1 Illustration of latent structure analysis. *Note* Q is yule's Q (Yule, 1912). This was used by lazarsfeld in his illustration 24
Fig. 2.2 Illustrative item response functions 25
Fig. 2.3 Path analysis (Wright, 1934, p. 161) 31
Fig. 2.4 Factor analysis (Thurstone, 1931, p. 100). *Note* Pitch discrimination (ability) is the latent variable 33
Fig. 2.5 Structural equation models with the LISREL model (Joreskog, 2007, p. 66). *Note* See Joreskog (2007) for a description of standard LISREL notation used for variables and arrows used in the model 35
Fig. 2.6 Graphical representations of the Rasch model. *Note* Adapted from wilson et al. (2008, p. 92) 37
Fig. 2.7 Graphical representation for three explanatory Rasch models. *Note* Dotted circle indicates random variable, Beta is fixed item effect, Z is random design effect, X is fixed design effect, and theta is random person effect. See text within the chapter for a deeper description 38
Fig. 2.8 Connections between invariance, measurement, and explanation 45
Fig. 3.1 Scatterplots for illustrative data with different dependent variables 52

Fig. 3.2	Simple linear model	53
Fig. 3.3	Wright Map. *Note* This version of a Wright Map was obtained in R using the EIRM package (Bulut, 2021)	61
Fig. 4.1	Definition of residuals	68
Fig. 4.2	Distribution of residual correlations	81
Fig. 4.3	Principal component analysis of residual correlations. *Note* Recommended critical value is 2.00—eigenvalues greater than 2.00 suggest additional potential dimensions in the residual correlations	82
Fig. 4.4	Item fit plots for learning stimulation scale	86
Fig. 4.5	Scatterplots of standardized residuals for selected items	87
Fig. 4.6	Scatterplots of standardized residuals for home 24 (misfitting, Outfit MSE = 2.00)	89
Fig. 5.1	Concept map for descriptive and explanatory models (dichotomous and polytomous data)	94
Fig. 5.2	Learning Stimulation Scale: Predicted probabilities for Item-Explanatory Rasch Model (Content Focus: Adult and Child Activities)	99
Fig. 5.3	Variable Map for ATC Scale. *Note* Variable Map was created using the Facets Program (Linacre, 1989)	100
Fig. 5.4	ATC Scale: Category Response Function (Rating Scale Model). *Note* The category probability functions were created using the Facets Program (Linacre, 1989)	105
Fig. 5.5	ATC Scale: Predicted probabilities for Item-Explanatory Rasch Model (Focus: Valence). *Note* −1 = Negative valence, 0 = Neutral valence, 1 = Positive valence	106
Fig. 5.6	ATC Scale: Predicted probabilities for Person-Explanatory Rasch Models (College and Gender)	108
Fig. 6.1	Principles for Invariant Rater-Mediated Assessments	115
Fig. 6.2	Illustrations of scoring designs for rater-mediated assessments	126
Fig. 6.3	Rater-mediated wright map for a descriptive RS-MFRM	131
Fig. 6.4	Examples of constant and non-constant adjustments for rater severity	139
Fig. 6.5	Scatterplots of standardized residuals for individual raters across domains	140
Fig. 6.6	Rater-mediated wright map with rater-specific threshold parameters	141
Fig. 6.7	Rater-mediated wright map with domain-specific threshold parameters	142
Fig. 6.8	Rater-mediated wright map for a person-explanatory PC-MFRM	143
Fig. 6.9	Illustrative category probability curves for a normal rater, central rater, and extreme rater	144

Fig. 6.10 Bivariate relationship between rater threshold SD and raters' use of central and extreme categories 145
Fig. 6.11 Contrast estimates for rater*subgroup interaction 146
Fig. 7.1 Five components for instrument development 158
Fig. 7.2 Sample construct map for transitive reasoning assessment 164
Fig. 7.3 Scatterplot of item difficulty parameters for transitive reasoning items from the Dichotomous Rasch model 168
Fig. 7.4 Histogram of student achievement parameters from the transitive reasoning assessment based on the Dichotomous Rasch model 169
Fig. 7.5 Wright map showing item and student parameter estimates from the transitive reasoning assessment based on the Dichotomous Rasch model 170
Fig. 7.6 Item covariate parameter estimates from the transitive reasoning assessment based on the LLRM 172
Fig. 7.7 Histogram of student achievement parameter estimates from the transitive reasoning assessment based on the LLRM 173
Fig. 7.8 Wright map showing item and student achievement parameter estimates from the transitive reasoning assessment based on the LLRM 174
Fig. 7.9 Construct map for biology exam 175
Fig. 7.10 Wright map showing item and student parameter estimates from the biology exam based on the Dichotomous Rasch Model 179
Fig. 7.11 Effects of cognitive demand and content for biology exam 181
Fig. 8.1 Illustration of recoded polytomous data using the EIRM package 192
Fig. 8.2 Plots of category probabilities for selected CESD items 198
Fig. 9.1 Principles for invariance 214

List of Tables

Table 1.1	Five principles of invariant measurement	2
Table 1.2	Rasch illustration of an ideal-type scale (Rasch, 1960/1980, pp. 65–66)	4
Table 1.3	Illustration of Guttman and Rasch item response patterns	5
Table 1.4	Summary of item calibrations for the learning stimulation scale	9
Table 2.1	Possible response patterns for four dichotomous items	19
Table 2.2	Guttman on the scaling of qualitative data	21
Table 2.3	Lazarsfeld on the translation of concepts into indices or scales	23
Table 2.4	Assumptions underlying mokken models for scaling	27
Table 2.5	Invariance and measurement	40
Table 2.6	Explanation and invariance	42
Table 3.1	Illustrative data for 10 persons	51
Table 3.2	Person by item matrix for learning stimulation scale (40 persons, 11 items)	55
Table 3.3	Wide to long format (5 persons, 4 items)	58
Table 3.4	Item calibrations for the learning stimulation scale	60
Table 4.1	Aspects of model-data fit	65
Table 4.2	Construct focus for learning stimulation scale	79
Table 4.3	Inter-item correlations of residuals: (aQ3)	80
Table 4.4	Summary statistics for dichotomous rasch model: Learning stimulation scale	85
Table 4.5	Summary statistics for items (Learning Stimulation Scale)	88
Table 4.6	Summary statistics for homes (Learning Stimulation Scale)	90
Table 5.1	First 10 cases for Learning Stimulation data files	94
Table 5.2	Estimates of item covariates (Learning Stimulation Scale)	98
Table 5.3	Attitude Toward Censorship scale	101
Table 5.4	ATC scale: Description of the participants	102
Table 5.5	First 10 cases for ATC scale files	102

Table 5.6 ATC scale: Model-data fit summary (Linear Logistic Rasch Models) 104
Table 5.7 Estimates of item covariates (ATC Scale) 106
Table 5.8 ATC scale: Model-data fit summary (Latent Regression Rasch Models) 107
Table 5.9 Estimates of person covariates (ATC Scale) 109
Table 6.1 Descriptive and explanatory many-facet Rasch Models 117
Table 6.2 Summary of parameter estimates and fit from descriptive MFRM-RS 137
Table 6.3 Summary of rater location estimates and fit from descriptive MFRM-RS 138
Table 6.4 Rater category use for Georgia writing data 147
Table 6.5 Differential rater functioning results for Georgia writing data 152
Table 7.1 Five components for instrument development 159
Table 7.2 Components for instrument development applied to the transitive reasoning assessment 163
Table 7.3 Transitive reasoning item classifications 164
Table 7.4 Components for instrument development applied to the biology exam 177
Table 7.5 Classification of biology Items by content domain and cognitive demand 178
Table 8.1 CESD item stems and classifications 189
Table 8.2 Illustration of polytomous recoding for GLMM estimation 190
Table 8.3 Indicators of rating scale functioning 194
Table 8.4 Average person location estimate (θ) within response categories for the CESD dataset 196
Table 8.5 Threshold ordering tests for the CESD items 197
Table 8.6 Average person location estimates within rating scale categories 204
Table 8.7 Rating scale threshold estimates for item classifications 204
Table 8.8 Average person location estimates within rating scale categories for education level groups 208
Table 8.9 Rating scale threshold estimates for item classifications 208

Chapter 1
Introduction

> *[Rasch Models] embody the essential principles of measurement itself, the principles on which objectivity and reproducibility, indeed all scientific knowledge are based*
> *(Wright, 1980, p. xix)*

Measurement theory is frequently defined by an apparent hodgepodge of psychometric models. In this book, the focus is on providing a coherent set of systematic guiding principles based on invariant measurement that allows the reader to understand what is arguably one of the essential aspects of modern science—the construction and use of scales to define the key constructs and variables that are essential for both theory and practice. Rasch measurement theory (Rasch, 1960/1980) offers a framework guided by scientific principles that can guide researchers in their efforts to construct, interpret, use, and improve scales across the human sciences. The human sciences include various disciplines, such as psychology, sociology, education, and economics, that define the social, behavioral, and health sciences in a broad way. Many of the guiding principles of measurement generalize across the sciences (Mari et al., 2021), but the focus of this book is on the unique problems faced in developing scales in the human sciences.

We provide an introduction to explanatory measurement models based on Rasch measurement theory that can be used to extend current views of measurement (De Boeck & Wilson, 2004). These extended models may include a set of predictors or covariates that can be used to explore relationships by combining measurement and explanation. These covariates can be used to expand our understanding of *why* items and persons vary in their locations on the latent variable being measured.

This chapter begins with an overview of Rasch measurement theory. Next, we briefly describe the Dichotomous Model proposed by Rasch (1960/1980) as a method that is widely used to develop psychometrically sound scales. Next, we introduce promising extensions to Rasch measurement theory models that include researcher-specified item and person covariates based on generalized linear mixed models. These explanatory Rasch models offer connections between measurement and explanation. The chapter ends with a discussion and summary of key points.

G. Engelhard and S. A. Wind, *Invariant Measurement with Explanatory Rasch Models in the Human Sciences*, https://doi.org/10.1007/978-3-032-08816-1_1

What is Rasch Measurement Theory?

> … contributions of the Danish mathematician and statistician Georg Rasch to social measurement can justifiably be called a measurement theory. (Andrich, 2018, p. 66)

Rasch measurement theory is one of the clearest examples of the application of scientific principles to achieve invariant measurement in the social and behavioral sciences. The basic principles of Rasch measurement theory can be stated in different ways. We have found it useful to summarize Rasch measurement theory in terms of five principles for invariant measurement to guide our thinking.

These five principles are shown in Table 1.1. The first principle is that the measurement process fosters the development of an invariant unidimensional scale. This implies that items and persons can be simultaneously located on a single underlying latent variable, represented visually as a line or linear continuum. Visual representations of the latent variable using a linear continuum have been called a variable map, item map, and Wright map. This is one of the key outcomes of Rasch measurement theory. It should be noted that the Wright Map was named in in honor of Benjamin D. Wright, who was a key figure in the enhancement and dissemination of Rasch's ideas.

The next principles are related to item-invariant measurement of persons, as well as person-invariant calibration of items. The item-invariant measurement of persons requires that the measurement of persons must be independent of the particular items that happen to be used for the measuring. It also implies that a more able person must always have a better chance of success on an item than a less able person (non-crossing person response functions). Person-invariant calibration of test items requires that the calibration of the items must be independent of the particular persons used for calibration. It also implies that any person must have a better chance of success on an easy item than on a more difficult item (non-crossing item response functions). Each of these principles are addressed in more detail in forthcoming chapters.

In this book, we develop a perspective on how to generalize these five principles for use with explanatory Rasch models. Chapter 2 gives a detailed discussion of

Table 1.1 Five principles of invariant measurement

Invariant unidimensional scale
1. Items and persons must be simultaneously located on a single underlying latent variable (Variable Map)
Item-invariant measurement of persons
2. The measurement of persons must be independent of the particular items that happen to be used for the measuring
3. A more able person must always have a better chance of success on an item than a less able person (Non-crossing person response functions)
Person-invariant calibration of test items
4. The calibration of the items must be independent of the particular persons used for calibration
5. Any person must have a better chance of success on an easy item than on a more difficult item (Non-crossing item response functions)

the principles related to invariance, measurement, and explanation guided by Rasch measurement theory. Chapter 2 also examines how these underlying principles relate to explanatory Rasch models that include a consideration of both measurement and explanation.

A useful starting point for developing an understanding of Rasch measurement theory is to consider ideal-type models. The German sociologist Max Weber described an epistemological perspective on the social sciences that stressed the utility of ideal-type models. Ideal-type models include direct statements about what is expected in observed data based on a theoretical perspective. The comparison between ideal and observed data provides a powerful analytic framework. Ideal-type models can include both deterministic and probabilistic models, as well as nonparametric and parametric models (Engelhard, 2013).

Rasch used an ideal-type approach as a starting point as shown in Table 1.2. Panel A (Table 1.2) presents his illustrative data set with 10 persons and 6 items, scored as correct (+) or incorrect (0). Panel B (Table 1.2) shows his suggestion to sort the data by item difficulty, defined using total scores. Panel C (Table 1.2) shows the data also sorted by item and person scores. These sorted matrices allow researchers to identify unexpected responses that do not match the overall expected order based on total scores. This procedure for identifying discrepancies between response patterns and total scores for persons and items reflects Guttman's (1944, 1950) approach to scaling, in which deviations from expected patterns are used to evaluate the scalability of item responses.

Although Rasch did not explicitly credit Guttman in suggesting these steps, Rasch's approach reflects defining Guttman scale patterns as an ideal type against which to evaluate observed responses. Whereas Guttman scaling principles can be viewed as deterministic, it is useful to view Rasch models as a probabilistic framework for evaluating Guttman patterns. Table 1.3 (Panel A) shows the distinctive triangular pattern of a Guttman scale that represents an ideal-type view of measurement. Rasch suggested a probabilistic version of this pattern that is illustrated in Table 1.2 (Panel B). Figure 1.2 shows the item response functions for both the Guttman Scale (Panel A), and the Rasch Scale (Panel B). It is important to note the stepwise form of the item response functions for the Guttman Scale that represents the deterministic and ideal-type characteristics of Guttman scales. Andrich (1985) provides a detailed account of the connections between Guttman and Rasch scaling. One of the consequences of viewing measurement in this way is that it highlights the elegance of Rasch measurement theory, but at the same time sets a high bar for approximating these ideal patterns for the scales used in the human sciences.

Rasch stressed the idea of invariant comparisons within a frame of reference as fundamental for science (Andrich, 2018; Stone & Stenner, 2014). Rasch (1960, pp. 331–332) proposed a set of principles for specific objectivity and invariant comparisons:

> The comparison between two stimuli should be independent of which particular individuals were instrumental for the comparison; and it should also be independent of which stimuli within the considered class were or might also have been compared.

Table 1.2 Rasch illustration of an ideal-type scale (Rasch, 1960/1980, pp. 65–66)

Panel A Original data matrix

person no.	item no. 1	2	3	4	5	6
1	+	+	o	+	o	+
2	o	o	o	+	o	o
3	+	+	+	+	+	+
4	o	+	o	+	o	o
5	+	+	+	+	+	+
6	+	+	o	+	o	+
7	+	+	o	+	+	+
8	o	o	o	o	o	o
9	+	+	o	+	+	+
10	o	+	o	+	o	o
number of correct answers to each item	6	8	2	9	4	6

Panel B Matrix sorted by items

person no.	item no. 4	2	1	6	5	3	number of correct items per person (raw score)
1	+	+	+	+	o	o	4
2	+	o	o	o	o	o	1
3	+	+	+	+	+	+	6
4	+	+	o	o	o	o	2
5	+	+	+	+	+	+	6
6	+	+	+	+	o	o	4
7	+	+	+	+	+	o	5
8	o	o	o	o	o	o	0
9	+	+	+	+	+	o	5
10	+	+	o	o	o	o	2

Panel C Matrix sorted by items and persons

person no.	item no. 4	2	1	6	5	3
3	+	+	+	+	+	+
5	+	+	+	+	+	+
7	+	+	+	+	+	o
9	+	+	+	+	+	o
1	+	+	+	+	o	o
6	+	+	+	+	o	o
4	+	+	o	o	o	o
10	+	+	o	o	o	o
2	+	o	o	o	o	o
8	o	o	o	o	o	o

Note Panel C reflects items sorted by item difficulty and persons sorted by sum scores. The triangular pattern of "+"s reflect an ideal Guttman pattern

> Symmetrically, a comparison between two individuals should be independent of which particular stimuli within the class considered were instrumental for the comparison; and it should also be independent of which other individuals were also compared on the same or on some other occasion

The first two principles in this list suggest that item calibrations (stimuli) should be invariant over the persons that are used to obtain the comparisons: person-invariant calibration of items. The last two principles suggest that person measurement should be invariant over the particular items (stimuli) that are used to obtain the comparisons: item-invariant measurement of persons.

One of the distinctive outcomes of Rasch measurement theory is the creation of a variable map. This map provides a visual representation of the latent variable that can be used to indicate the locations of both persons and items on a continuum. When the principles for invariant measurement are met, person locations are invariant across items, and item locations are invariant across persons. As a result, researchers can

Table 1.3 Illustration of Guttman and Rasch item response patterns

Panel A	Guttman (deterministic)					
	Item					
Person	1	2	3	4	5	6
A	1	1	1	1	1	0
B	1	1	1	1	0	0
C	1	1	1	0	0	0
D	1	1	0	0	0	0
E	1	0	0	0	0	0
Panel B	*Rasch (probabilistic)*					
A	0.98	0.95	0.75	0.65	0.50	0.40
B	0.95	0.75	0.65	0.45	0.40	0.35
C	0.75	0.65	0.45	0.34	0.25	0.20
D	0.65	0.45	0.35	0.25	0.20	0.10
E	0.50	0.35	0.25	0.15	0.10	0.05

Note Guttman patterns are deterministic and Rasch patterns are probabilistic

use variable maps as a concise and coherent summary of a latent variable. Figure 1.1 provides a generic example of a variable map. Typically, these maps only include person and item locations. In Fig. 1.1, we have included a preview of how extended Rasch models can be used to structure item and person characteristics by grouping persons into two categories and grouping items into two classifications. The use of both person and item classifications (i.e., designs) represent extensions to Rasch measurement theory that include covariates to predict person and item locations.

Andrich (2018) made a strong case for viewing Rasch's contributions to measurement as a *theory of measurement* rather than simply a set of Rasch models. In his words, "contributions of Rasch in articulating a case for invariant comparisons as fundamental to generalizable knowledge, and rendering these in the form of probabilistic models that can be used for a range of derivations of new insights and applications, constitute a measurement theory and therefore justifies being referred to as Rasch Measurement Theory" (p. 88). We describe Rasch's philosophy of measurement and elaborate on his views relative to invariant measurement in more detail in Chap. 2.

Dichotomous Model

In order to be concrete regarding Rasch measurement theory, we start here with the Dichotomous Model proposed by Rasch (1960/1980). The Dichotomous Model can be used to illustrate the underlying principles of Rasch measurement theory. The simplest case is to imagine a person responding to a set of achievement test items that

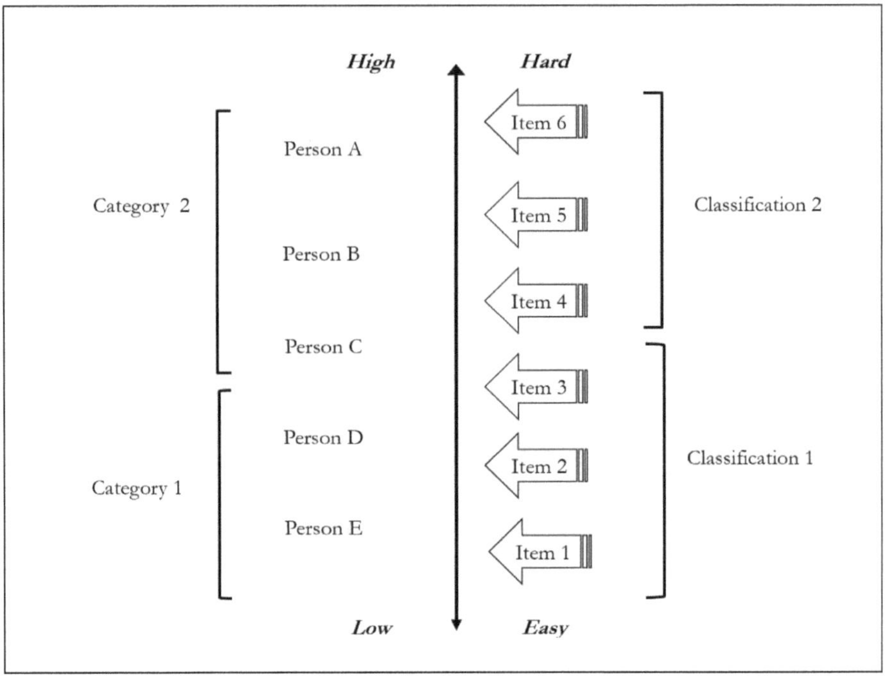

Fig. 1.1 Generic variable map. *Note* Categories indicate subgroups of persons (e.g., male/female), while classifications indicate subsets of items (e.g., adult-/child-dominated activities)

can be scored dichotomously (0 = incorrect, 1 = correct). Reflecting on measurement in the physical sciences, Rasch hypothesized that ideally only two components should influence the probability of a correct response to a test item: (1) the location of the item and (2) the location of the person on the underlying continuum. The comparison between the item and person locations should determine the probability of a correct response. If a person and item share the same locations, then the probability of a correct answer is 0.50. If a person's location is above the item location, then the probability is greater than 0.50. Conversely, if a person's location is below the item location, the probability of a correct answer is less than 0.50. Rasch selected a logistic response model to represent this relationship between probability of a correct answer as a function of the distance between the person and items.

The Dichotomous Model can be written as the probability of a positive response:

$$P(X_{ni} = 1) = \frac{\exp(\theta_n - \delta_i)}{1 + \exp(\theta_n - \delta_i)} \tag{1.1}$$

where θ_n is location of person n on the latent variable, and δ_i is the location of item i on the latent variable. Figure 1.2 (Panel B) shows the item response functions for the Dichotomous Model with three persons ($\theta = -2, 0, 2$). In the figure, person locations are shown on the x-axis, and the probability for a response is shown on the y-axis. These item response functions (IRFs) illustrate the probabilistic relationship between person locations and item responses that characterize Rasch models. The Dichotomous Model is important to aid in understanding the modeling of polytomous data addressed later in the book.

The Dichotomous Model can also be written in logit (log odds) format as

$$\eta_{ni} = ln\left[\frac{P(X_{ni} = 1)}{1 - P(X_{ni} = 1)}\right] \tag{1.2}$$

and

$$\eta_{ni} = \theta_n - \delta_i \tag{1.3}$$

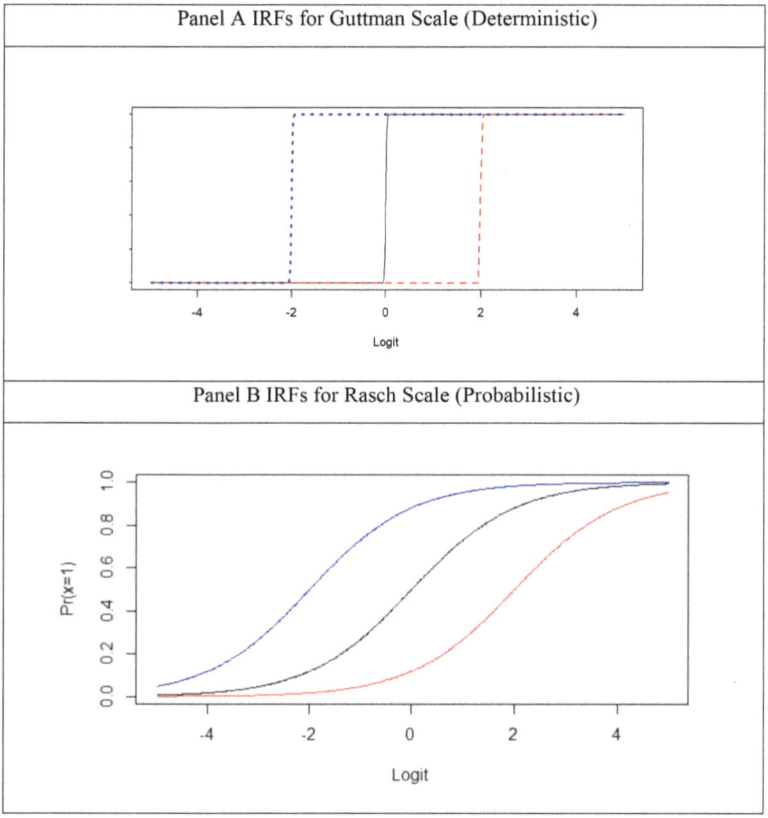

Fig. 1.2 Three item response functions (IRFs) for Guttman and Rasch Scales with three persons (θ = −2, 0, 2)

The Dichotomous Model is also known as Rasch's simple logistic model (Andrich, 1988). This representation in terms of logits provides a key for estimating Rasch models using generalized linear mixed models.

Illustration

In practice, researchers can use the Dichotomous Model to explore measurement instruments from the perspective of invariance. For example, the Learning Stimulation Scale was developed to define aspects of learning stimulation in home environments for preschool children (Engelhard, 2013). There are 11 items and 40 homes in this data set. In this application, homes are interpreted like persons (i.e., examinees) in the Dichotomous Model, and a theta estimate (θ) is calculated for each home. Table 1.4 describes the items included in the Learning Stimulation Scale. Table 1.4 also includes item location estimates on the logit scale (δ) obtained for the original calibration of the items based on the Dichotomous Model, where the estimates have been scaled such that the average location estimate equals zero. Table 1.4 includes the original calibrations based on joint maximum likelihood estimation, as well as item calibrations obtained from the TAM (Robitzsch et al., 2021) and eirm (Bulut, 2021) packages in R. Both TAM and eirm use marginal maximum likelihood estimation as the default estimation procedure.

Figure 1.3 provides the variable map for a scale designed to measure learning stimulation in the home. This Learning Stimulation Scale summarizes item and person estimation results from the Dichotomous Model. The first column is the logit scale, the second column indicates the location of the home environments, ordered from low to high learning stimulation, and the third column indicates the item locations on the scale. For items, higher locations suggest that an activity was rare—these activities were only observed in homes with high levels of learning stimulation. Lower locations suggest that activities were readily observed in homes that did not necessarily stimulate learning. The fourth column indicates item groups that reflect the degree to which an item relates primarily to adult-dominated or child-dominated activities. This fourth column is simply a label at this point, but it will be included in future analyses as a part of an explanatory Rasch model.

Researchers can use the results in Fig. 1.3 to consider the characteristics of homes as environments for stimulating learning. For example, activities that are related to children were observed more readily than activities related to adults.

Explanatory Rasch Models

The Dichotomous Model has been extended in several ways that allow researchers to explore important characteristics of latent variables beyond item difficulty and person locations. Useful extensions to the Dichotomous Model include the Linear

Table 1.4 Summary of item calibrations for the learning stimulation scale

			Original calibration (Engelhard, 2013)		TAM calibration		EIRM calibration	
Item number	Item	Focus	Item location	Standardized	Item location	Standardized	Item location	Standardized
1	Toys (color size and shape)	Child	−1.71	−0.93	−1.52	−0.97	−2.58	−0.93
2	Puzzles	Adult	1.33	0.73	1.20	0.76	0.14	0.73
3	Music player	Adult	1.97	1.08	1.76	1.12	0.71	1.08
4	Toys (free expression)	Child	−2.47	−1.35	−2.21	−1.41	−3.26	−1.34
5	Toys (refined movements)	Child	0.57	0.31	0.51	0.32	−0.55	0.31
6	Toys (teach numbers)	Child	−1.14	−0.62	−1.02	−0.65	−2.08	−0.62
7	Ten or more children's books	Child	0.08	0.04	0.07	0.04	−1.00	0.04
8	Ten books visible	Adult	0.41	0.22	0.37	0.24	−0.70	0.22
9	Newspaper	Adult	1.64	0.90	1.48	0.94	0.42	0.90
10	Magazine	Adult	2.32	1.27	2.06	1.31	1.01	1.26
11	Shape learning	Child	−3.01	−1.64	−2.71	−1.73	−3.76	−1.65
Mean			0.00	0.00	0.00	0.00	−1.06	0.00
SD			1.83	1.00	1.57	1.00	1.64	1.00

Note Item focus indicates that the classification of an item emphasizes either child or adult-dominated activities. Original calibration is based on joint maximum likelihood, while TAM (Robitzsch et al., 2021) and EIRM (Bulut, 2021) are based on marginal maximum likelihood estimation. It should be noted that TAM and EIRM can estimate item locations as item difficulty (as shown here) or as item easiness

```
+------------------------------------------------+
|Logit|+Homes                     |-Items|-Focus|
|-----+---------------------------+------+------|
|   4 + 1  9  28             High + Hard +      |
|     |                           |      |      |
|     |                           |      |      |
|     |                           |      |      |
|     |                           |      |      |
|     | 6  8  27 34 39            |      |      |
|   3 +                           +      +      |
|     |                           |      |      |
|     |                           |      |      |
|     |                           |      |      |
|     | 4  15 25 29 31            | 10   | A    |
|     |                           |      |      |
|   2 +                           + 3    + A    |
|     |                           |      |      |
|     | 3  23 40                  | 9    | A    |
|     |                           |      |      |
|     |                           | 2    | A    |
|     |                           |      |      |
|   1 + 2  5  10 11 12 18 22 30 38 +      +      |
|     |                           |      |      |
|     |                           |      |      |
|     |                           | 5    | C    |
|     | 13 14 17 24 32 35 37      | 8    | A    |
|     |                           |      |      |
*   0 *                           * 7    * C    *
|     | 16 20                     |      |      |
|     |                           |      |      |
|     |                           |      |      |
|     |                           |      |      |
|     | 21                        |      |      |
|  -1 +                           +      +      |
|     |                           | 6    | C    |
|     |                           |      |      |
|     | 7  26                     |      |      |
|     |                           | 1    | C    |
|     |                           |      |      |
|  -2 +                           +      +      |
|     |                           |      |      |
|     | 19 33 36                  |      |      |
|     |                           | 4    | C    |
|     |                           |      |      |
|     |                           |      |      |
|  -3 +                           + 11   + C    |
|     |                           |      |      |
|     |                           |      |      |
|     |                           |      |      |
|     |                           |      |      |
|     |                           |      |      |
|  -4 +                       Low + Easy +      |
|-----+---------------------------+------+------|
```

Fig. 1.3 Variable map for learning stimulation scale. *Note* Home data (40 homes, 11 items, focus of activities: A = adult-dominated activities, and C = child-dominated activities)

Logistic Rasch Model (LLRM) and the Latent Regression Rasch Model (LRRM). We discuss and explore these models extensively in this book.

The original family of Rasch models also included extensions for polytomous models (Wright & Masters, 1982). The most common polytomous Rasch models are the Partial Credit Model (Masters, 2016) and the Rating Scale Model (Andrich, 2016). These models have also been extended to include rater effects with the Facets Model (Linacre, 1989).

It is also possible to extend the family of Rasch models further using Generalized Linear Mixed Models (GLMMs), which are Generalized Linear Models (GLMs) with random effects; this approach provides researchers with a great deal of flexibility in specifying models to incorporate item and person characteristics. In their general applications, researchers use GLMs to transform categorical dependent variables using a linking component (e.g., logistic function) to provide a framework for using well-known regression and ANOVA models. The motivation for using GLMs is that researchers can apply linear statistical models with various researcher-specified independent variables to situations where the dependent variable is categorical, such as scored dichotomous or polytomous responses to assessments or survey instruments. Tutz (2011), Faraway (2016), and Pinheiro and Bates (2006) provide helpful general introductions to GLMs and GLMMs.

In the context of Rasch measurement theory, researchers have considered how the GLMM approach can be used to define and estimate Rasch models, including extended Rasch models (de Boeck et al., 2011). Using a GLMM approach to present and define these models, De Boeck and Wilson (2004) refer to measurement models without covariates as descriptive models, and measurement models with covariates as explanatory models. In Chap. 3, we present a detailed discussion of the use of GLMMs to estimate Rasch measurement models. As a preview, we can use a GLMM format to write the linear logistic extension of the Dichotomous Model that includes item covariates as:

$$\eta_{ni} = \theta_n - \sum_{k=1}^{K} \beta_k X_{ik} \tag{1.4}$$

where θ_n is a random effect for persons, β_k is a fixed effect for items, and X_{ik} is a design matrix for defining item characteristics, such as item types. For example, the Learning Stimulation Scale has two types of items that focus on adult or child activities. In the LLRM, the β_k parameters reflect the average difficulties associated with each item classification (adult- or child-dominant items). This model has also been called the linear logistic test model (LLTM; Fischer, 1973).

Table 1.4 includes the calibrations of the items estimated with a generalized linear mixed model (GLMM) for the Dichotomous Model. The standardized versions of the original item locations and the GLMM estimates are essentially the same as in the Dichotomous Model analysis, but the results now include item characteristics in addition to overall item difficulty. The learning stimulation data set is revisited in future chapters.

Discussion and Summary

This chapter has introduced several key ideas that are developed throughout the book.

A major goal of this book is to develop a conceptualization of invariant measurement that can be used to develop, estimate, and interpret explanatory Rasch models. Rasch measurement theory is not simply defined by a particular family of measurement models that are labeled with Rasch's name. Rasch measurement theory is defined by scientific principles based on the concept of specific objectivity and invariance applied to models of measurement. Rasch measurement theory offers an approach for progress in research that has implications for measurement and statistics, as well substantive theory and practice in the human sciences.

Rasch measurement theory represents a key paradigm shift in measurement. van der Linden (2016) has suggested that the first chapter of Rasch's book is required reading for anyone seeking to understand the transition from classical test theory to item response theory. In his words, "One of the best introductions to this change of paradigm [from classical or traditional test theory] is Rasch (1960/1980, Chapter 1), which is mandatory reading for anyone with an interest in the subject" (p. xvii).

It is interesting that other paradigm shifts in the history of measurement have been related to advances in statistical modeling. Statistical advances often provided new perspectives on how to address measurement issues. For example, Classical Test Theory is dependent in a fundamental way on the use of correlation coefficients (Clauser, 2022; Spearman, 1904a, 1904b, 1910), Generalizability Theory was developed around the use of Analysis of Variance (Cronbach et al., 1972; Hoyt, 1941), and Item Response Theory is strongly related to the use of logistic regression models (Luecht & Hambleton, 2022; Rasch, 1960/1980). The use of GLMMs offers the measurement community the potential for similar advances regarding the development of new models, as well as conceptual and substantive insights into a variety of measurement issues.

In summary, Rasch measurement theory has frequently been presented as a set of stand-alone models that are not tied to other statistical modeling frameworks. In this book, we argue that it is useful to view Rasch models within the broader statistical framework of GLMMs. Considering Rasch models from the perspective of GLMMs allows researchers to understand connections between these models and other statistical approaches. This perspective facilitates the extension of Rasch models in interesting and useful ways.

References

Andrich, D. (1985). An elaboration of Guttman scaling with Rasch models for measurement. In N. B. Tuma (Ed,), *Sociological methodology* (pp. 33–80). Jossey-Bass.

Andrich, D. (1988). *Rasch models for measurement*. Sage Publications, Inc., Id.

Andrich, D. (2016). Rasch rating-scale model. In W. J. van der Linden. (Ed.), *Handbook of item response theory, volume 1: Models* (pp. 75–94). CRC Press.

Andrich, D. (2018). A Rasch measurement theory. In F. Guillemin, A. Leplege, S. Briancon, E. Spitz, & J. Coste (Eds.), *Perceived health and adaptation in chronic disease* (pp. 66–91). Routledge.

Bulut, O. (2021). *EIRM: Explanatory item response modeling for dichotomous and polytomous item responses [Computer software].* http://CRAN.R-project.org/package=EIRM

Clauser, B. (2022). A history of classical test theory. In B. Clauser & M. Bunch (Eds.), *History of educational measurement in the United States* (pp. 157–180). Routledge.

Cronbach, L. J., Gleser, G. C., Nanda, H., & Rajaratnam, N. (1972). *The dependability of behavioral measurements: Theory of generalizability for scores and profiles.* Wiley.

De Boeck, P., Bakker, M., Zwitser, R., Nivard, M., Hofman, A., Tuerlinckx, F., & Partchev, I. (2011). The estimation of item response models with the lmer function from the lme4 package in R. *Journal of Statistical Software, 39*, 1–28.

De Boeck, P., & Wilson, M. (Eds.). (2004). *Explanatory item response models: A generalized linear and nonlinear approach.* Springer.

Engelhard, G. (2013). *Invariant measurement: Using Rasch models in the social, behavioral, and health sciences.* Routledge.

Faraway, J. J. (2016). *Extending the linear model with R: Generalized linear, mixed effects and nonparametric regression models.* Chapman and Hall/CRC.

Fischer, G. H. (1973). The linear logistic test model as an instrument in educational research. *Acta Psychologica, 37*(6), 359–374.

Guttman, L. (1944). A basis for scaling qualitative data. *American Sociological Review, 9*(2), 139–150.

Guttman, L. (1950). The basis for scalogram analysis. In S. A. Stouffer, L. Guttman, E. A. Suchman, P. F. Lazarsfeld, S. A. Star, & J. A. Clausen (Eds.), *Measurement and prediction* (Vol. IV, pp. 60–90). Princeton University Press.

Hoyt, C. J. (1941). Test reliability estimated by analysis of variance. *Psychometrika, 6*, 153–160.

Linacre, J. M. (1989). *Many-facet Rasch measurement.* MESA Press.

Luecht, R. M., & Hambleton, R. K. (2022). Item response theory: A historical perspective and brief introduction to applications. In B. Clauser & M. Bunch (Eds.), *History of educational measurement in the United States* (pp. 232–262). Routledge.

Masters. (2016). Partial credit model. In W. J. van der Linden (Ed.), *Handbook of item response theory, volume 1: Models.* (pp. 109–126). CRC Press.

Mari, L., Wilson, M., & Maul, A. (2021). *Measurement across the sciences: Developing a shared concept system of measurement.* Springer.

Pinheiro, J., & Bates, D. (2006). *Mixed-effects models in S and S-PLUS.* Springer.

Rasch, G. (1960/1980). *Probabilistic models for some intelligence and attainment tests.* Danish Institute for Educational Research (Expanded edition, Chicago: University of Chicago Press, 1980).

Robitzsch, A., Kiefer, T., & Wu, M. (2021). *TAM: Test analysis modules. R package version 3.7-16.*

Spearman, C. E. (1910). Correlation calculated from faulty data. *British Journal of Psychology, 3*, 271–295.

Spearman, C. E. (1904a). The proofs and measurement of association between two things. *American Journal of Psychology, 15*, 72–101.

Spearman, C. E. (1904b). "General intelligence" objectively determined and measured. *American Journal of Psychology, 15*, 201–293.

Stone, M. H., & Stenner, A. J. (2014). Comparison is key. *Journal of Applied Measurement, 15*(1), 26–39.

Tutz, G. (2011). *Regression for categorical data.* Cambridge University Press.

van der Linden, W. J. (Ed.). (2016). *Handbook of item response theory, volume 1: Models.* CRC Press.

Wright, B. D., & Masters, G. N. (1982). *Rating scale analysis: Rasch measurement.* MESA Press.

Chapter 2
Measurement, Explanation, and Invariance

Measurement and explanation are not mutually exclusive. (De Boeck & Wilson, 2016, p. 567)

In Chap. 1, we briefly introduced explanatory Rasch models as tools with which researchers can explore and explain relationships between variables in a measurement context. In this chapter, we take a step back from technical aspects of these models to consider the theoretical relationship between *explanation* and *measurement*, and how this relationship provides a foundation for creating, using, and evaluating explanatory Rasch models. Our discussion emphasizes and connects three major themes: (1) invariance, (2) measurement, and (3) explanation. This chapter develops these three themes and their connections.

The first section of this chapter explores the concept of invariance and its implications for measurement theory. To explore the connections between measurement and invariance, we consider in detail the measurement theories of Guttman (1944, 1950), Lazarsfeld (1950a, 1950b, 1960, 1968), Mokken (1971, 1997), and Rasch (1960/1980,1961, 1964, 1977). Next, we discuss the relationship between explanation and invariance with implications for examining structural relationships that underlies science broadly conceived (Godfrey-Smith, 2003; Nozick, 2001; Woodward, 2000, 2021). For the purposes of this book, we focus on four general perspectives on explanation: path analysis (Wright, 1934), factor analysis (Spearman, 1904; Joreskog, 2007; Thurstone, 1935, 1947), structural equation modeling (Bollen, 1989; Joreskog, 2007), and explanatory item response models (De Boeck and Wilson, 2004, 2016). We selected these perspectives to guide our thinking about invariant structural relationships and Rasch measurement theory. The final section considers how measurement, invariance, and explanation can be combined to create a set of basic guiding principles for explanatory Rasch models.

G. Engelhard and S. A. Wind, *Invariant Measurement with Explanatory Rasch Models in the Human Sciences*, https://doi.org/10.1007/978-3-032-08816-1_2

Invariance and Measurement

> The mathematical rendition of the requirements of invariance in a probabilistic framework ... is the major contribution to Rasch's work having the characteristics of a theory (Andrich, 2018, p. 79).

The philosopher Robert Nozick (1998, 2001) identified invariance as an essential feature of science related to the concept of objectivity. Nozick (1998, 2001) described four specific and related aspects of objectivity. First, evidence for objectivity is provided by accessibility from different perspectives. When something is objective, it is accessible by different observers, and objectivity can be replicated under different conditions. The second aspect of objectivity is intersubjectivity. This implies independent agreement among observers. The third aspect relates to independence. Objectivity is evident when it is independent of the particular beliefs, desires, and hopes of observers. Finally, the fourth aspect relates to invariance, which underlies all of the other aspects of objectivity. According to Nozick (2001),

> what is objective about something, I have claimed, is what is invariant from different angles, across different perspectives, and under different transformations. Yet often what is variant is what is especially interesting. We can take different perspectives on a thing (the more angles the better), and notice which of its features are objective and invariant, and also notice which of its features are subjective and variant. (p. 102)

Measurement plays a foundational role in all sciences. An early statement of this perspective is that "the history of science is the history of measurement" (Cattell, 1893, p. 316). A similar view of the importance of measurement is echoed in the twenty-first century:

> It would be difficult to overstate the value and importance of measurement in nearly every aspect of society. Every time we purchase or eat food, take prescribed medicine, travel in a vehicle, use a phone or computer, or step inside a building, we place our trust int the results of measurement—and for the most part, that trust seems well earned, and as such measurement is commonly associated with precision, accuracy, and overall trustworthiness. (Mari et al., 2021).

Measurement theories are conceptual models that provide a systematic way to understand, evaluate, and interpret assessment processes. One popular view of measurement is based on Stevens who stated that "measurement, in the broadest sense, is defined as the assignment of numerals to objects or events according to rules" (Stevens, 1946, p. 677). Of course, this definition does not define the specific rules that are embedded within different measurement theories. The three research traditions (test score, scaling, and structural traditions) discussed later in this chapter highlight groupings of measurement models with different characteristics. This book focuses on the using the concept of invariance as the underlying principle underlying several measurement theories. Although different measurement theories provide various perspectives on invariance, this book focuses on Rasch measurement theory as a broad framework in which to develop, apply, and evaluate the measures or scales that have been developed to represent a latent variable or construct. Essentially, the "rules" come from the quest for invariance within the context of Rasch measurement theory.

Measurement theories play an important role in so many aspects of our lives because they:

- define the aspects of quantification that are defined as problematic,
- determine the statistical models and appropriate methods used to solve these problems,
- determine the impact of our research in the social, behavioral and health sciences,
- frame the substantive conclusions and inferences that we draw, and ultimately
- delineate and limit the policies and practices derived from our research work in the social, behavioral and health sciences (Engelhard, 2013, p. 80)

Given the ubiquitous aspects of measurement, it is important to consider the basic principles that guide our evaluations of how well our measures are functioning. It is also important to broaden these principles beyond traditional indices of psychometric quality to include a consideration of structural relationships among scales.

Numerous measurement theorists have emphasized connections between invariance and measurement. For example, several measurement theorists have discussed requirements for invariance, including Thorndike (1904), Thurstone (1959), Guttman (1944, 1950), Lazarsfeld (1950), Mokken (1971, 1997), and Rasch (1960/1980, 1961, 1964, 1977). These measurement theorists have important connections related to how they conceptualize measurement with regard to invariance, among other issues. In a series of publications, Engelhard (1984, 1991, 1992, 1994, 2013) discussed and compared these measurement theorists' perspectives related to key measurement concepts, including invariance. Focusing on these four key measurement theorists, we organize our thinking around three issues that have implications for invariance in measurement: (1) construct (latent variable), (2) person measurement, and (3) item calibration. Our main goal in considering these four theorists in detail is to clarify common issues or themes, and to lay the groundwork for generalizing these issues into principles to guide evaluation of invariant structural relationships in the next section.

The first major connection between our selected theorists is that their measurement theories emphasize the central role of a single unidimensional construct or latent variable. A second issue that cuts across measurement theories is the idea that person measurement should be independent or invariant over different sets of items. The third issue is that item calibrations and procedures for locating items on the latent variable representing the construct should be independent of particular persons. These three issues can be briefly described as follows:

- Construct (Latent Variable): Items and persons must be simultaneously located on a unidimensional underlying continuum
- Person Measurement: The measurement of persons must be independent of the particular items used (Item-invariant measurement of persons). A more able person must always have a better chance of success on an item than a less able person.

- Item Calibration: The calibration of the items must be independent of the particular persons used (Person-invariant calibration of test items). Any person must have a better chance of success on an easy item than on a more difficult item.

Guttman

> One of the fundamental problems facing research workers ... is to determine if the questions asked on a given issue have a single meaning for the respondents. Obviously, if a question means different things to different respondents, then there is no way that the respondents can be ranked ... Questions may appear to express a single thought and yet not provide the same kind of stimulus to different people. (Guttman, 1950, p. 60)

In the 1940s, Louis Guttman (1944, 1950) laid the groundwork for a new technique designed to explore the unidimensionality of a set of items. Guttman proposed a set of requirements that can be used to test the hypothesis of unidimensionality. Guttman Scaling or Scalogram Analysis is the specific technique he recommended for determining the degree to which a set of items and group of persons meet the requirements of a Guttman Scale. Guttman Scales are also called perfect scales (Engelhard, 2005).

Guttman determined the requirements of a unidimensional scale based on the idea that an underlying continuum can be used to represent a latent variable or construct. Guttman scales can be defined and visualized in several ways. If we start with a data matrix (persons by items), then the requirements of Guttman scaling are met when person scores are sufficient to reproduce the exact pattern of item responses in the data matrix. In his words,

> [a] particularly simple representation of the data would be to assign to each individual a numerical value and ... given the value of the individual and the values of the categories of an attribute, we could reproduce the observations of the individual on the attribute. (Guttman, 1944, p. 143)

Guttman scales yield "an unambiguous meaning to the order of scale scores ... within each item" (Guttman, 1950, p. 89). Guttman sought a method for person measurement based on a person's score that reflected an ideal pattern of item responses based on ordered items. In Guttman's words,

> [i]f a person endorses a more extreme statement, he should endorse all less extreme statements if the statements are to be considered a scale ... We shall call a set of items of common content a scale if a person with a higher rank than another person is just as high or higher on every item than the other person. (Guttman, 1950, p. 62)

When persons and items are ordered and displayed in a table, then the data matrix forms a distinctive triangular pattern for a perfect Guttman scale. This pattern is shown in the top panel of Table 2.1 (Panel A). The person scores are listed in descending order (4 to 0), and the items are ordered from easy to hard (A is easy ... D is hard). It should be noted that person scores assigned to each response pattern exactly identify the specific items that the person answered correctly or incorrectly.

No information is lost by replacing item response patterns with person scores. For example, a person with a score of 3 and a perfect response pattern is expected to respond correctly to the three easiest items (A, B, and C), and incorrectly to the hardest item (D). A four-item test composed of dichotomous items has 16 possible response patterns ($2^4 = 16$). There are five perfect response patterns, and eleven imperfect patterns ("Guttman errors"). The eleven imperfect patterns are shown in the bottom panel of Table 2.1 (Panel B).

Guttman items can be represented with item response functions that show the relationship between the latent variable on the x-axis, and the probability of answering the item positively on the y-axis. Panel A in Fig. 2.2 shows item response functions for four Guttman items. Guttman items are modeled as deterministic (rather than probabilistic) with a distinctive step pattern: For each item, there is a person score beyond which a correct response is always observed.

Table 2.1 Possible response patterns for four dichotomous items

Index		Panel A Perfect Guttman Patterns			
	Person Scores	A	B	C	D
1	4	1	1	1	1
2	3	1	1	1	0
3	2	1	1	0	0
4	1	1	0	0	0
5	0	0	0	0	0
		Panel B Imperfect Patterns			
	4	None			
6	3	1	1	0	1
7	3	1	0	1	1
8	3	0	1	1	1
9	2	1	0	1	0
10	2	0	1	1	0
11	2	1	0	0	1
12	2	0	1	0	1
13	2	0	0	1	1
14	1	0	1	0	0
15	1	0	0	1	0
16	1	0	0	0	1
	0	None			

Note Four dichotomous items yield 16 response patterns (24 = 2 x 2 x 2 x 2). Items are ordered from easy (Item A) to hard (Item D). There are five perfect Guttman patterns, and 11 imperfect Guttman patterns

Two other ideas are important for understanding Guttman's theoretical perspective on scaling: a universe of attributes (items, questions), and a population of objects (persons). First, Guttman (1944) defines the universe of attributes as follows:

> the universe is the concept whose scalability is being investigated ... The universe consists of all the attributes that define the concept ... it consists of all of the attributes of interest to the investigation which have a common content. (Guttman, 1944, p. 141)

Guttman makes clear that items must have common content if they are to be used to define a unidimensional scale, and that these items should be viewed as sampled from a larger universe of potential items that define the construct or latent variable. If the requirements of a Guttman scale are achieved, then invariant scaling of persons is possible regardless of the particular sample of items used to rank-order the persons. This idea of sampling from a larger domain of content is important when random item effects are included in measurement models; we discuss this idea further later.

Guttman's second major concept clarifies his view of a population of objects (persons). Guttman points out that the persons used for scaling should be purposely selected according to well-defined criteria. Guttman (1944) suggests that an "investigator must always delimit the population of objects or individuals with which he is working" (p. 142). Guttman was worried that the scalability of a set of items may not be invariant over different groups of persons. This becomes a very important issue because if the items are not invariant over groups, then it is not possible to compare them. In Guttman's words,

> if a universe is scalable for one population but not for another population or forms a scale in a different manner, we cannot compare the two populations in degree and say that one is higher or lower on the average than another with respect to the universe. (Guttman, 1944, p. 150)

Guttman's emphasis on well-defined populations reflects a concern with sample-invariant item calibration across groups. This idea appears within modern measurement in the form of differential item functioning or measurement invariance (Millsap, 2011). This idea connects to generalized linear mixed models when person covariates are included in the analyses.

Table 2.2 summarizes the basic steps in the creation of a Guttman scale in an extensive quote. Guttman scaling can be used to create a unidimensional scale to represent a latent variable with person scores that define a specific pattern of item responses. Guttman's view of item calibration emphasized person-invariant item calibrations by sampling from a domain of potential items or indicators of the latent variable. Guttman also suggested that a scale may not function in the same way for different groups of persons, and that it is important to identify the limits and context of generalization. As we demonstrate later in this chapter, this perspective on generalization is similar to Rasch's (1960/1980, 1977) idea of specific objectivity.

Table 2.2 Guttman on the scaling of qualitative data

SUMMARY

1. The multivariate frequency distribution of a universe of attributes for a population of objects is a scale if it is possible to derive from the distribution a quantitative variable with which to characterize the objects such that each attribute is a simple function of that quantitative variable.
2. There is an unambiguous meaning to the order of scale scores. An object with a higher score than another object is characterized by higher, or at least equivalent, values on each attribute.
3. There is an unambiguous meaning to the order of attribute values. One category of an attribute is higher than another if it characterizes objects higher on the scale.
4. It can be shown that if the data are scalable, the orderings of objects and of categories are in general unique (except for direction). Both orderings emerge from analysis of the data, rather than from *a priori* considerations.
5. The predictability of any outside variable from the scale scores is the same as the predictability from the multivariate distribution with the attributes. The zero order correlation with the scale score is equivalent to the multiple correlation with the universe. Hence, scale scores provide an invariant quantification of the attributes for predicting any outside variable whatsoever.
6. Scales are relative to time and to populations. a. For a given population of objects, a universe may be scalable at one time but not at another, or it may be scalable at two periods of time but with different orderings of objects and categories. b. A universe may be scalable for one population but not for another, or it may be scalable for two populations but with different orderings of objects and categories. c. Comparisons with respect to degree can be made only if the same scaling obtains in both cases being compared.
7. From the multivariate distribution of a sample of attributes for a sample of objects, inferences can be drawn concerning the complete distribution of the universe for the population. a. The hypothesis that the complete distribution is scalable can be adequately tested with a sample distribution. b. The rank order among objects according to a sample scale is essentially that in the complete scale. c. The ordering of categories in a sample scale is essentially that in the complete scale.
8. Perfect scales are not found in practice. a. The degree of approximation to perfection is measured by a coefficient of reproducibility, which is the empirical relative frequency with which values of the attributes do correspond to intervals of a scale variable. b. In practice, 85 percent perfect scales or better have been used as efficient approximations to perfect scales.
9. In imperfect scales, scale analysis picks out deviants or non-scale types for case studies.

Guttman (1944, p. 150)

Lazarsfeld

> [W]e always have the task of making inferences from a variety of manifest indicators as to the underlying or intended characterization of the object under investigation— its latent characteristics. (Lazarsfeld, 1955, p. 392)

Paul Lazarsfeld was a sociologist who made several significant contributions to quantitative methodology, including important advances in measurement (1960, 1966, 1968). In particular, his measurement work on latent structure analysis introduced the concept of local independence. The basic idea of latent structure analysis is that the observed relationships between items is due to an underlying latent variable, and if this latent variable is held constant (i.e., partialled out), the probability of responding positively to two or more items is equal to the product of the probabilities of responding positively to each item. This principle of local independence undergirds much of the modern work on item response theory (Baker & Kim, 2004; Lazarsfeld & Henry, 1968).

Latent structure analysis is the mathematical formulation of what Lazarsfeld (1955) called a "diagnostic process" (p. 392). According to him, the goal of measurement is the classification of people using underlying latent properties based on a variety of indicators or items. Latent structure analysis is the mathematical framework used to support "inferences from a variety of manifest indicators as to the underlying or intended characterization of the object under investigation— its latent characteristics" (Lazarsfeld, 1955, p. 392).

In thinking about measurement, Lazarsfeld (1968) identified four steps for scale construction: Reflection on the initial "imagery," concept specification, selection of indicators, and the formation of scales and indices. Table 2.3 includes a long quote that describes in detail how Lazarsfeld viewed these four steps. The first two steps support the important problem of how to develop the concept of a latent variable. The third step of concept specification provides a way of expanding the meaning of the latent variable based on underlying components. It should be stressed that these components are similar to the classifications used in tables of specifications or test blueprints for achievement tests. The fourth step of indicator selection includes the concept of interchangeability. Lazarsfeld (1955) suggests that invariance of person scores can occur over different subsets of items selected to represent the latent variable.

Lazarsfeld developed latent structure analysis to mathematically connect observed indicators (e.g., item responses) to the underlying latent variable (construct). Latent structure analysis bears several commonalities with test theory, and Lazarsfeld (1960) points out that "latent structure analysis can be looked upon as a generalization of test theory models" (p. 84). Latent structure analysis is also closely related to some of the foundational principles of factor analysis, including the idea of latent variables or factors. As pointed out by Stouffer (1950), the "latent structure approach is a generalization of Spearman-Thurstone factor analysis" (p. 19) to qualitative data. This connection was also noted by Bartholomew (2007).

Lazarsfeld's view of latent variables and how to discover them using latent structure analysis is one of his singular achievements in measurement. To illustrate the concept of local independence, Lazarsfeld starts with the simple idea that a population can be created by mixing two separate groups of persons. In order to illustrate his idea, he used the relationship between two dichotomously scored items (Items 1 and 2). Lazarsfeld used Yule's Q to measure the association between the two items within each group (Yule, 1912), and this statistic has a similar interpretation to other correlational indices with values of -1.00 to $+1.00$ indicating strength and direction of the association. Figure 2.1 shows how observed data with two groups (A and B) with no association between item responses (Yule's $Q = 0$) can be combined to form a new group (Combined) with an association of Yule's $Q = .58$. The key feature of this example with observed data is that the two items that are not related in either Groups A or B, can be combined into a group that exhibits an association between the two items.

Table 2.3 Lazarsfeld on the translation of concepts into indices or scales

[The] process by which concepts are translated into empirical indices has four steps: an initial imagery of the concept, the specification of dimensions, the selection of observable indicators, and the combination of indicators into indices.

1. Imagery. The flow of thought and analysis and work which ends up with a measuring instrument usually begins with something which might be called imagery. Out of the analyst's immersion in all the detail of a theoretical problem, he creates a rather vague image or construct. The creative act may begin with the perception of many disparate phenomena as having some underlying characteristic in common. Or the investigator may have observed certain regularities and is trying to account for them. In any case, the concept, when first created, is some vaguely conceived entity that makes he observed relations meaningful … This kind of general impression starts the wheels rolling for a measurement problem.
2. Concept Specification. The next step is to take this original imagery and divide it into components. The concept is specified by an elaborate discussion of the phenomena out of which it emerged. We develop "aspects", "components", "dimensions", or similar specifications. They are sometimes derived logically from the overall concept, or one aspect is deduced from another, or empirically observed correlations between them are reported. The concept is shown to consist of a complex combination of phenomena, rather than a simple and directly observable item.
3. Selection of Indicators. After we have decided on these dimensions, there comes the third step: finding indicators for the dimensions. Here, we run into a number of problems. First of all, how does one "think up" indicators? The problem is an old one.
4. Formation of Indices. In the formation of indices of broad social and psychological concepts, we typically select a relatively small number of items from a large number of possible ones suggested by the concept and its attendant imagery. It is one of the notable features of such indices that their correlation with outside variables will usually be about the same, regardless of the specific "sampling" of items which goes into them from the broader group associated with the concept. This rather startling phenomenon has been labeled "the interchangeability of indices".

Lazarsfeld (1958, pp. 101-105)

Note Quotation marks in the original

In latent structure analysis, the process is essentially reversed. In Fig. 2.1, latent structure analysis is used to separate (i.e., "un-mix") the combined data of observed data into two latent groups (α and β) where the two items are unrelated within each group. The key idea is that if the relationship between the two items disappears, then this latent variable is viewed as an explanatory variable that accounts for the relationship that appears in the combined group.

Figure 2.2 (Panel B) shows the item response functions ("trace lines" in his words) for four Lazarsfeld items. Contrasting this with Guttman's deterministic item response functions, Lazarsfeld's items are modeled to be probabilistic with no common parametric form across items for the relationship between the latent variable and the probability of a positive response.

In practice, the underlying latent variable is unknown, and the task is to find local independence after controlling for the latent variable. Latent structure analysis is the general name for models that have been proposed for unmixing qualitative data. It is beyond the scope of this chapter to describe in detail how this unmixing occurs,

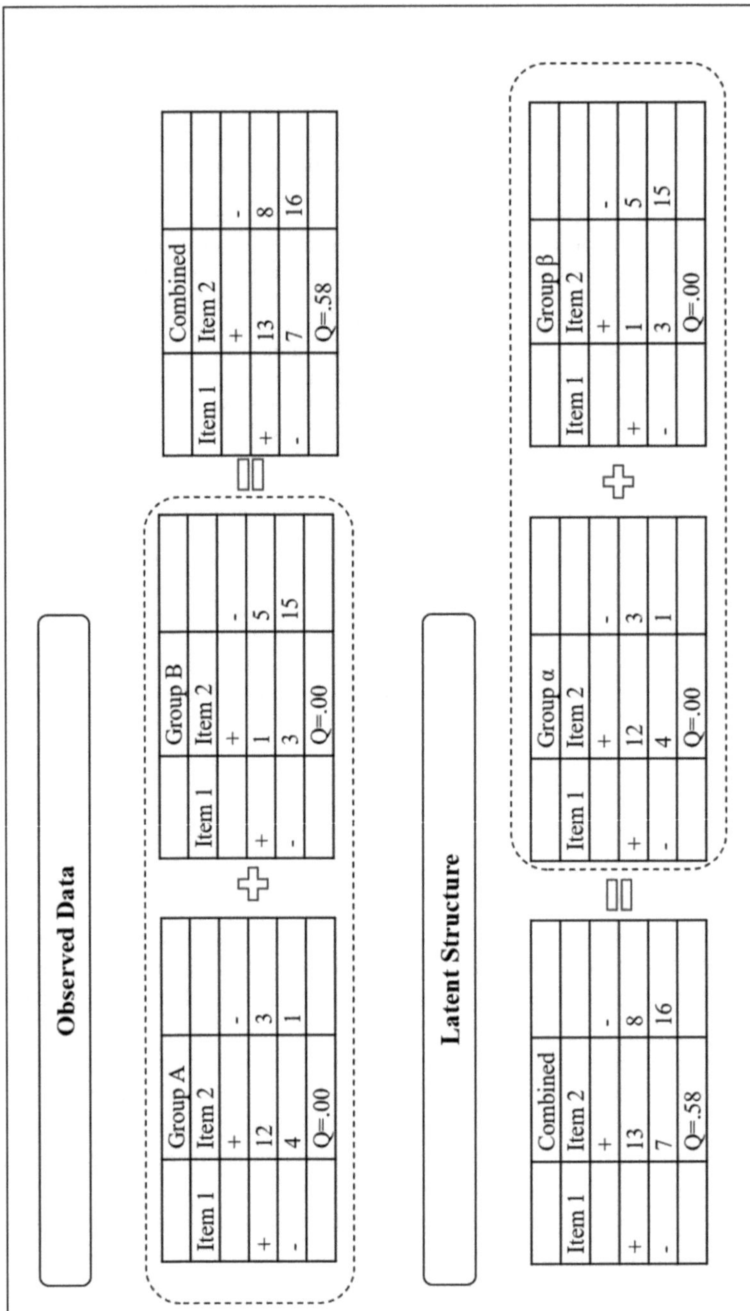

Fig. 2.1 Illustration of latent structure analysis. *Note* Q is yule's Q (Yule, 1912). This was used by lazarsfeld in his illustration

a: Guttman Items Guttman-Scaling Model	b: Lazarsfeld Items (1955, p. 396) Latent-linear Model
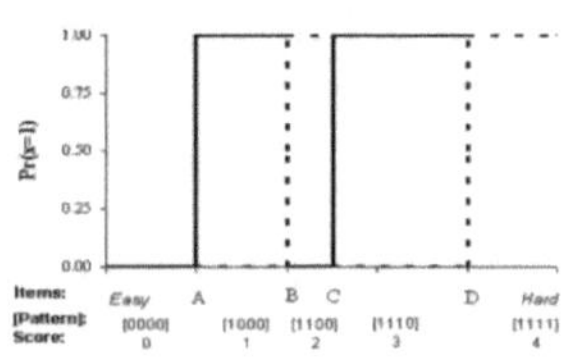	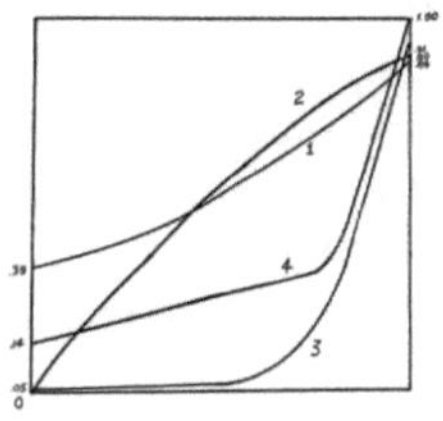
c: Mokken Items: Monotone-Homogeneity Model (Sijtsma & Molenaar, 2002, p. 14)	d: Mokken Items: Double-Monotonicity Model (Mokken, 1997, p. 355)
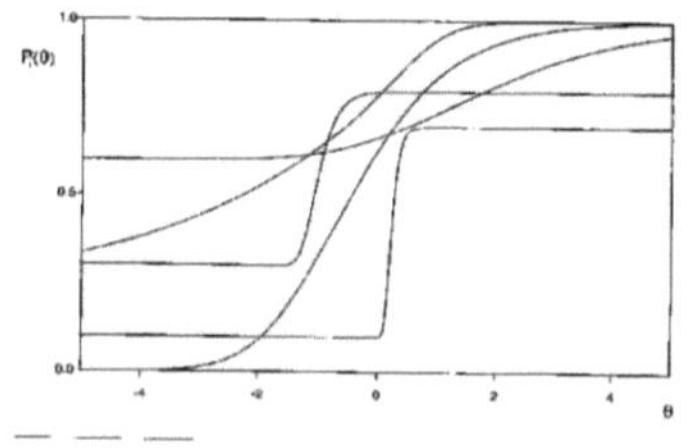	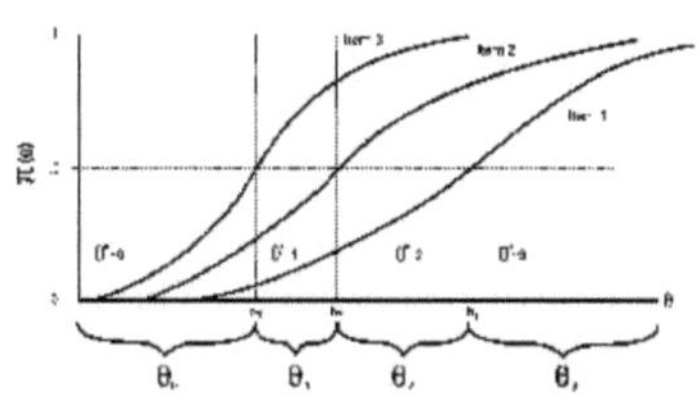
e: Rasch Items (1960/1980, p. 71)	f: Rasch Items (Wright, 1997, p. 42)
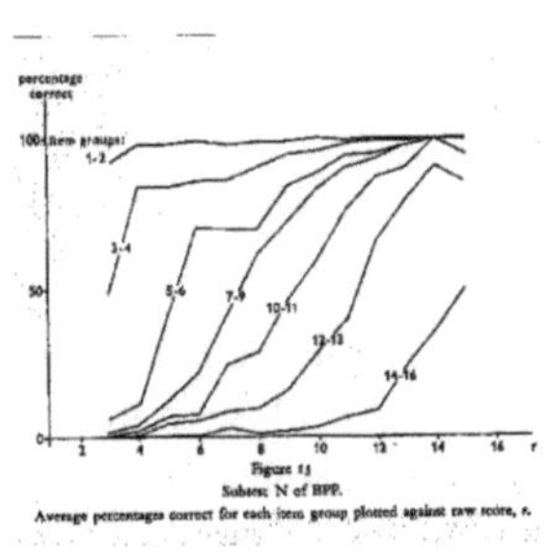	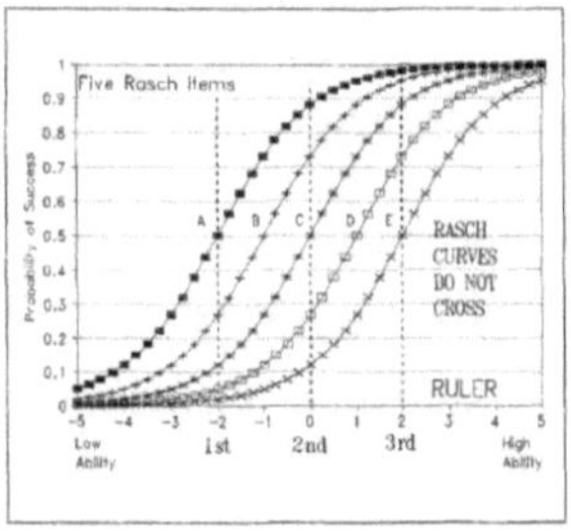

Fig. 2.2 Illustrative item response functions

and Lazarsfeld and Henry (1968) provide the computational details about how to use latent structure analysis.

Mokken

> Scaling procedures of the type we are looking for may be based on such general assumptions as monotone homogeneity and holomorphism (double monotonicity), and the manifest (observable) properties which result from these assumptions only. (Mokken, 1971, p. 176)

Mokken was a political scientist who developed an approach to scaling. His models can be viewed as nonparametric item response models for the unidimensional scaling of dichotomous items (Mokken, 1971, 1997; Mokken & Lewis, 1982; Sijtsma & Molenaar, 2016; Wind, 2017). Mokken scaling is a bridge between Guttman scaling (deterministic and nonparametric model) and Rasch measurement theory (probabilistic and parametric models) with some connections to concepts introduced by Lazarsfeld (1959).

Mokken (1971) sought a new approach to item response modeling because he felt that:

> in vast areas of social research the application of parametric models may often be too far-fetched. Their application presupposes a relatively deep insight into the structure of the variable to be measured and the properties of the items by which it can be measured . . . [and] lead to procedures of inference and estimation that are too pretentious and intricate for the level of information and the precision that can be claimed for the data used in actual measurement. (p. 173)

Mokken (1971) identified for four assumptions to guide the development of practical scales for researchers. The four assumptions underlying Mokken scaling are as follows:

1. Unidimensionality: Item responses reflect evidence of a single latent variable.
2. Local Independence: Responses to an item are not influenced by responses to any other item, after controlling for the latent variable.
3. Monotonic Response Functions: The probability of a positive response is nondecreasing across increasing values of the latent variable (monotone homogeneity).
4. Nonintersecting and Monotonic Item Response Functions: Items order persons in a similar way, and persons order items in a similar way (double monotonicity).

The first assumption is unidimensionality. As with the other scaling models in this section, Mokken (1971) sought to create unidimensional scales. In his words, "The position of an individual is reduced to one value, which indicates his position (score) on the single dimension, the interpretation of which again depends on the problem behind the data" (Mokken, 1971, p. 13).

Mokken's second important assumption is related to local independence. As pointed out earlier, local independence was introduced by Lazarsfeld (1959). It can be defined as the assumption that for a person with a given location on the latent variable, the responses to a set of items are statistically independent (no association) conditional on the person's location. This assumption underlies all item response theory approaches (Baker & Kim, 2004).

The third assumption is that the item response functions are monotonically nondecreasing functions of the latent variable. This is shown in Fig. 2.2 (Panel C). Mokken called this property monotone homogeneity (MH). Mokken (1977) introduced a related property called "similar ordering" that "reflects the possibility of a unidimensional representation of the persons in terms of an ability supposed to underlie their response behavior" (p. 353). Similar ordering and monotone homogeneity are equivalent properties with similarity ordering properties emphasizing support for the unidimensionality of the scale. A set of items that meets the MH condition can be used to provide an ordering of persons on the latent variable. In practice, Mokken models use sum scores to define the latent variable, and this yields an ordinal scale supported by a monotonically non-decreasing set of items in the scale.

The fourth assumption is double monotonicity (DM). This assumption includes the idea that item response functions must be nonintersecting and monotonically non-decreasing. This is shown in Fig. 2.2 (Panel D). The first three assumptions are essential for the ordering of persons on the latent variable. The DM assumption adds the requirement of uniform ordering of items. In other words, MH requires that items order persons in a similar way, while DM adds the condition that persons should also order items in a similar way.

Mokken introduced two models characterized by these assumptions. The first is the Monotone Homogeneity (MH) model that meets assumptions one to three, and the second is the Double Monotonicity (DM) model that meets all four of the assumptions. The MH model can be used to create an invariant ordering of persons based on a set of items that meet the first three assumptions. For the DM model, both invariant person and item ordering can be obtained if the items fit the model. Table 2.4 shows the relationship between the MH and DM models related to these four assumptions. Essentially, the MH model is based on the first three major assumptions, while DM model adds the fourth assumption. Mokken scales yield person scores on an ordinal scale (rank ordering).

The two Mokken models can also be illustrated using item response functions. Panel C in Fig. 2.2 illustrates Mokken items based on the MH model, while Panel D in Fig. 2.2 illustrates the DM model.

It is important to note that the assumptions of Mokken scaling are similar to the requirements of Rasch measurement theory. The Rasch model meets the requirements of the DM model. The main difference is that Mokken scaling yields ordinal measures, while Rasch models yield metric measures (Rost, 2001). Mokken models are nonparametric with sum scores used to define the latent variable. The Rasch model also uses the sum score as a sufficient statistic to define an interval scale when good model-data fit is obtained.

Table 2.4 Assumptions underlying mokken models for scaling

	Monotone Homogeneity Model	Double Monotonicity Model
Latent variable	1. Unidimensionality 2. Local independence	1. Unidimensionality 2. Local independence
Person measurement	3. Monotonically non-decreasing IRFs	3. Monotonically non-decreasing IRFs
Item calibration		4. Monotonically increasing non-crossing IRFs

Rasch

The concept of "objectivity" raises fundamental problems in all sciences. For a statement to be scientific, "objectivity" is required. (Rasch 1964, p. 1)

Rasch's goal was to develop models for measurement that supported "individual-centered statistical techniques in which each individual is characterized separately and from which, given adequate data, the individual parameters can be estimated" (Rasch, 1960/1980, p. xx). To accomplish this goal, Rasch started with a perspective on science that included the concept of objective comparisons. In his words (Rasch, 1964):

Looking then for concepts [of measurement] that could possibly be taken as primary it seems worth-while to concentrate upon two essential characteristics of "scientific statements":

1. they are concerned with "comparisons" [and]
2. the statements are claimed to be "objective" [quotes in the original] (p. 2)

As pointed out earlier by Nozick (2001), objectivity in scientific statements depends on several features including accessibility, intersubjectivity, independence, and most importantly, invariance that implies the first three characteristics. These four features of objectivity in science can be applied to measurement processes.

Rasch identified objective comparisons as a key concept in science, as well as in measurement. Rasch defined objective comparisons as follows:

> The comparison between two stimuli [items] should be independent of which particular individuals were instrumental for the comparison; and it should also be independent of which other stimuli [items] within the considered class were or might also have been compared.
>
> Symmetrically, a comparison between two individuals should be independent of which particular stimuli [items] within the class considered were instrumental for the comparison; and it should also be independent of which other individuals were also compared, on the same or on some other occasion. (Rasch, 1977, pp. 331–332)

Rasch recognized the importance of identifying the conditions under which objective comparisons are invariant. He also introduced the idea of specific objectivity that stresses that invariance may not occur under all conditions. He argued for the importance of specifying a frame of reference to delineate the conditions for invariant measurement. This emphasis echoes Nozick's (2001) suggestion that it is important to notice both objective and invariant features, as well as to "notice which of its features are subjective and variant" (p. 102).

Invariant and variant features are two sides of the same coin in the sense that establishing invariance includes an exploration of sources of variance that may place limits on the consistency and generalizability of the measuring process. For example, in the measurement of temperature, researchers do not expect all instruments to function across the full range of temperatures (Chang, 2004)—we would use a different thermometer to measure a child's fever as compared to the temperature of molten steel. It is also important to note that the search for variant aspects implies anomalies that play a key role in the history of science (Andrich, 2002; Kuhn, 1970).

Rasch measurement theory is strongly related to the other measurement theories discussed in this section. Rasch models embody many of the characteristics of probabilistic Guttman scales (Andrich, 1985). Rasch measurement theory is also strongly related to latent structure analyses (Lazarsfeld, 1959). Rasch measurement theory has many characteristics in common with the double monotonicity model of Mokken scaling with the additional characteristic of yielding a metric scale (Rost, 2001).

The empirical item response functions are shown in Fig. 2.2 (Panel E) presented by Rasch (1960/1980). Four Rasch items are shown in Fig. 2.2 (Panel F) presented by Wright (1997). Rasch items are modeled to be probabilistic with logistic form of the relationship between the latent variable and the probability of a positive response.

Rasch developed a philosophy of measurement that included the application of basic scientific concepts including objectivity and invariance. Rasch measurement theory represents scientific principles based on the concept of specific objectivity (invariant comparisons) applied to models for measurement. Rasch measurement theory aims to create invariant scales and provide objective measures.

In the next section, we turn our attention to several perspectives on explanation and invariance in science that has the potential to unite the concepts of measurement, explanation, and invariance.

Explanation and Invariance

> Science aims at the discovery … of relationships that are invariant under some large or relevant range of circumstances. (Woodward, 2021, p. 267)

Explanation plays a key role in science (Godfrey-Smith, 2003). A major aim of science is to describe the structure of the world. Science also aims to explore why things happen. Although philosophers of science may disagree, it is our perspective that science has a strong explanatory role in addition to its descriptive role. Measurement is a key aspect of science that does not merely describe latent variables—it also plays a role in explaining relationships among variables.

Woodward (2000, 2021), who is a philosopher of science, has made a strong case for the connections between explanation and invariance. His philosophical perspective provides an opportunity for extending the principles of invariance to explore relationships between variables. According to Woodward (2000), "explanatory relationships are relationships that in principle can be used for manipulation and control in the sense that they tell us how certain (explanandum) variables would change if other (explanans) variables were to be changed or manipulated" (p. 198). He also stresses that the utility of an explanation depends on the degree and domain of invariance. In his words,

> A generalization is invariant if (i) it is … change-relating and (ii) it is stable or robust in the sense that it would continue to hold under a special sort of change called an intervention. (Woodward, 2000, p. 198)

Woodward (2000) argued that relationships between two or more variables are invariant if they continue to hold as other conditions vary. The changes over which the relationships are invariant define a domain of invariance. Invariance is a relative matter and includes the identification of the frames of reference under which relationships are stable and consistent. It is also important to note that degrees of invariance may hold. Measuring instruments may not function in the same way under all conditions. In other words, invariance is not an all or nothing matter because generalizations may be invariant under some interventions and not invariant under others. The concept of domain invariance suggested by Woodward (2000) is similar to Rasch's concept of specific objectivity and frames of reference (Rasch, 1977).

In relating the ideas of measurement and structural analyses, Engelhard and Wang (2024) identified three measurement traditions that can be used to organize our thinking about theories of measurement with connections to structural relationships: test score, scaling, and structural traditions. The test score tradition includes Classical Test Theory and Generalizability Theory. The main focus is on the reduction of measurement error. The second tradition is the scaling tradition, which includes all of the measurement theories discussed in previous section including Guttman, Lazarsfeld, Mokken, and Rasch. Measurement theories in the scaling tradition focus on the creation of an invariant continuum to represent a latent variable or construct. Finally, the structural tradition considers connections between science and measurement more generally. The structural tradition seeks to identify invariant relationships between variables.

In this section, we consider the structural tradition in detail. We present structural ideas using several approaches that are not typically related to measurement issues. We believe that there are essential connections between measurement and structural analyses. We selected these structural approaches because of their implications for connecting explanation and invariance to measurement broadly conceived. The specific approaches to structural relationships discussed in this section include:

- path analysis (Duncan, 1966; Wright, 1921, 1934),
- factor analysis (Spearman, 1904; Thurstone, 1947),
- structural equation modeling (Bollen, 1989; Joreskog, 1969), and
- explanatory item response models (De Boeck & Wilson, 2004).

Path Analysis

> The method of path coefficients [is] a flexible means of relating the correlation coefficients between variables in a multiple system to the functional relations among them. (Wright, 1934, p. 161)

Path analysis was developed by Sewall Wright (1921, 1934). One of the key aspects of path analysis that is relevant for our purposes is the graphical displays used to represent relationships among variables. Path diagrams provide a useful system for representing relationships among several variables. Strictly speaking, path analysis is not a measurement model. However, like other structural approaches, it explores functional relationships among a set of variables. In addition to path diagrams, current uses of path analysis include the decomposition of covariance and correlations in terms of path model parameters with an important distinction between direct and indirect effects (Bollen, 1989). Path analysis also has important conceptual links to current views regarding causal inferences in the social sciences (Pearl, 2018).

An early depiction of a path analysis model is shown in Fig. 2.3 (Wright, 1934). In this case, we see many of the conventions that are used today for path diagrams (Pastor & Finney, 2015). V_0 on the far right is the dependent variable and it is directly influenced by V_1 and V_2 as shown by a single-headed arrow pointing to V_0. V_u is viewed as a residual effect on V_0. V_1 and V_2 are directly influenced by V_4, V_5, and V_6. Wright (1934) proposed a series of rules for estimating path coefficients for a set of variables based on their correlation matrix. Path analysis is an early example of structural analyses among variables based on correlations that anticipated many current approaches including structural equation modeling. In fact, path analyses can be described as structural equations with observed variables.

Since the focus of path analysis is on relationships among observed variables reflected in correlation matrices and path diagrams, measurement issues were not directly considered in early research. This is perhaps because Wright conducted this early work within the field of genetics, which did not have the same measurement problems as those encountered in the human sciences. Wright (1934) used both unstandardized and standardized variables with appropriate cautions regarding interpretation of the resulting path coefficients. Connecting this approach to a measurement context, Bond et al. (2020) point out that the observed variables can be replaced

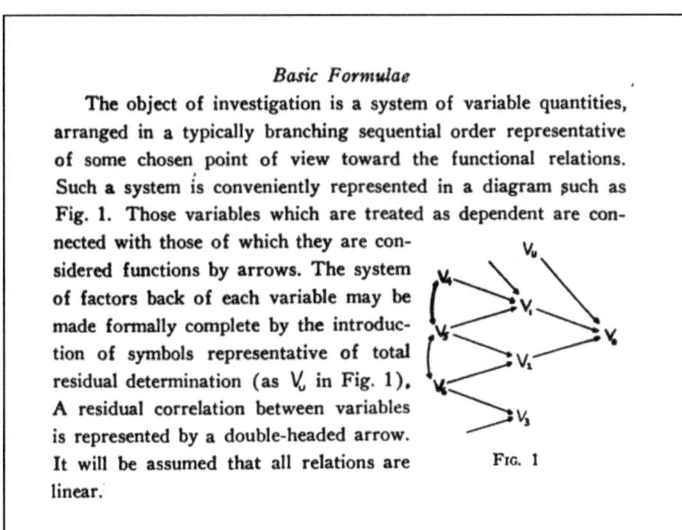
Basic Formulae

The object of investigation is a system of variable quantities, arranged in a typically branching sequential order representative of some chosen point of view toward the functional relations. Such a system is conveniently represented in a diagram such as Fig. 1. Those variables which are treated as dependent are connected with those of which they are considered functions by arrows. The system of factors back of each variable may be made formally complete by the introduction of symbols representative of total residual determination (as V_u in Fig. 1). A residual correlation between variables is represented by a double-headed arrow. It will be assumed that all relations are linear.

Fig. 2.3 Path analysis (Wright, 1934, p. 161)

with Rasch calibrated person scores (θ), and then included in a path analysis model to support explanatory research within a measurement framework.

We use conceptual aspects of path analysis to inform our views on structural relationships that are relevant to defining invariant measurement and relationships. Path diagrams provide useful roadmaps to guide our thinking about substantive aspects of research in the human sciences. Path analysis has several implications for our thinking about explanatory Rasch models. By focusing on diagrams, our substantive thinking is made visible regarding relationships among variables. It also supports our view of scientific activities that includes both description and explanation.

Factor Analysis

> The primary goal [of factor analysis] is to explain the covariances or correlations between many observed variables by means of relatively few underlying latent variables. (Bollen, 1989, p. 226)

Factor analysis was developed as way of identifying underlying latent variables or factors. Spearman (1904) is credited with inventing factor analysis based on the idea that the correlations between a set of tests designed to measure human abilities could be represented by a latent factor or variable that he called *g*. Spearman's methodology was based on partial correlations (Bollen, 1989). Thurstone (1931, 1947) also contributed significantly to the methodology of factor analysis through his introduction of multiple factor analysis. Figure 2.4 shows a graphical representation of a factor analysis created by Thurstone (1931). In this case, the latent variable is auditory pitch discrimination, and the four observed variables include two teachers' estimates of pitch discrimination, as well as two objective tests. It is interesting to note that Thurstone's diagram did not include arrow heads to indicate directionality.

As pointed out by Joreskog (2007), developments in the 1950s led factor analysis to be defined as a statistical method (Lawley & Maxwell, 1971). This fostered the view of factor analysis as a data reduction method. It also disconnected factor analysis as a method from the earlier controversies related to the measurement of intelligence and eugenics (Gould, 1996).

Factor analysis has fostered several important ideas that are relevant for this book. One important idea is the distinction between exploratory and confirmatory factor analysis. As its name implies, exploratory factor analysis (EFA) is used to identify the underlying relationships between observed variables using factors (latent variables) that are not hypothesized before the analysis. EFA is frequently used to evaluate the dimensionality of an observed set of data. This is particularly important because item response models, including Rasch models, require unidimensionality, and this requirement can be evaluated with factor analysis.

Confirmatory factor analysis (CFA) is another relevant idea that can be used to evaluate whether the data fit a hypothesized model (Joreskog, 1969). In CFA, the constraints are based on specified hypotheses that force the model to be consistent

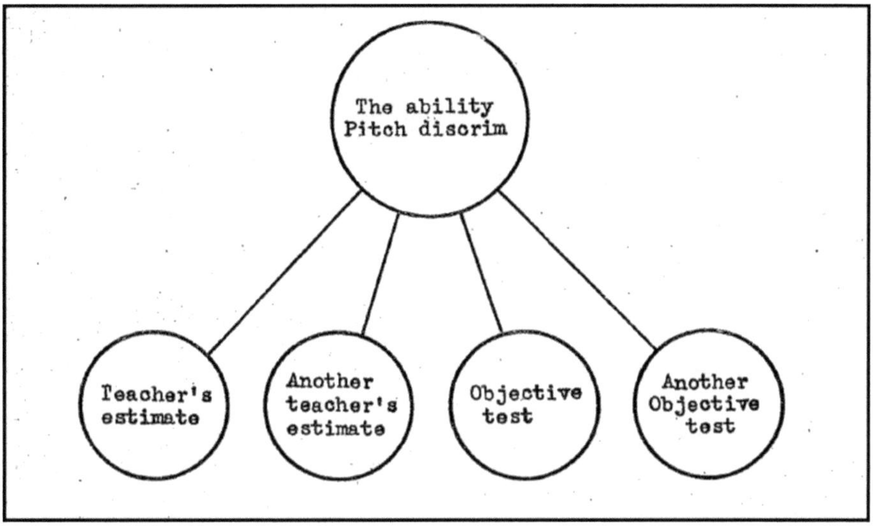

Fig. 2.4 Factor analysis (Thurstone, 1931, p. 100). *Note* Pitch discrimination (ability) is the latent variable

with an underlying theory. In measurement, item response models can be viewed as confirmatory factor analysis models. Factor loadings have a close relationship to the slope or discrimination parameters included in the two-parameter logistic model (Baker & Kim, 2004). From a factor-analytic perspective, Rasch models require factor loadings to be fixed to be equal to 1 or another constant. In examining model-data fit, factor-analytic methods are utilized along with other methods in Chap. 4.

Factor-analytic solutions have several indeterminacies that can lead to multiple ways of modeling a data set. The concept of *simple structure* was proposed by Thurstone (1947) as one method for addressing indeterminacies related to factor rotation. Basically, simple structure is a guiding principle for finding psychologically meaningful factors. The general idea of simple structure is that if the factors have real psychological meaning, then items will have clear loadings on distinct factors (Joreskog, 1966). Thurstone (1947) specified several conditions for simple structure that "enables us to obtain an invariance of factorial description" (p. 181). An important point is that Thurstone (1947) introduced a closely related concept that he called factorial invariance. In his words, "the factorial description of a test must remain invariant when the test is moved from one battery to another which involves the same common factors" (Thurstone, 1947 p. 361).

Thurstone's concept of factorial invariance was developed in more detail by Meredith (1993). Meredith (1993) identified several aspects of factorial invariance including configural invariance, strong factorial invariance, strict factorial invariance, and weak measurement invariance. Millsap (2011) systematically extended these aspects of factorial invariance and provided a general approach for examining measurement invariance more broadly. Measurement invariance is closely related to differential item functioning (Holland & Wainer, 1993). The concept of invariance used in this book goes beyond measurement invariance to encompass aspects of invariance related to both items and persons, as well as invariant relationships.

It should be noted that factor analysis and latent structure analysis are both built on similar conceptualizations of latent variables (Bartholomew, 2007). Factor analysis in its traditional form focuses on the reproduction of a matrix of correlations or covariances between a set of test scores based on a smaller number of underlying factors or latent variables (Bollen, 1989). Latent structure analysis on the other hand, focuses on contingency tables reflecting relationships between categorical data (Lazarsfeld & Henry, 1968).

The main implications of factor analysis for this book include the distinction between explanatory and confirmatory analyses, the concept of factorial invariance, and the close connections between factor analysis, latent structure analysis, and item response theory. Mulaik (1986) provides a detailed history of the major developments in factor analysis with an emphasis on structural aspects. The edited volume by Cudeck and MacCallum (2007) provides multiple perspectives on the history of factor analysis.

Structural Equation Modeling

> After a set of factors has been identified, it is natural to go on and use the factors themselves as predictor or outcome variables in further analyses. Broadly speaking, this is the goal of structural equation modeling. (Joreskog, 2007, p. 62)

Structural equation modeling combines aspects of both measurement (factor analysis) and analyses of relationships (covariance analysis) between observed and latent variables (Bollen, 1989; Joreskog, 1969). As discussed in the previous section, factor analysis forms the basis for the measurement model, while path analysis and regression models provide the structural equation aspects of the model. Factor analysis can be used to identify underlying latent variables or factors, and then these latent variables can be used in the structural equations.

Structural equation models (SEMs) provide a very general approach for data analysis. It is important to recognize that SEMs are not modeling individual observations, but the emphasis is on "covariances rather than cases" (Bollen, 1989, p. 1). As was the case for other structural approaches, SEMs provide graphical displays that aid the conceptualization of the relationships between both observed and latent variables or factors.

Joreskog (2007) proposed a general model called LISREL which is an abbreviation of linear structural relations. Figure 2.5 shows an example of the diagrams used with the LISREL models (Joreskog, 2007). See Joreskog (2007) for a description of standard LISREL notation for variables and arrows used in this example.

Because standard applications of SEMs are based on factor analysis as the measurement model, there are several limitations of SEMs as implemented in social

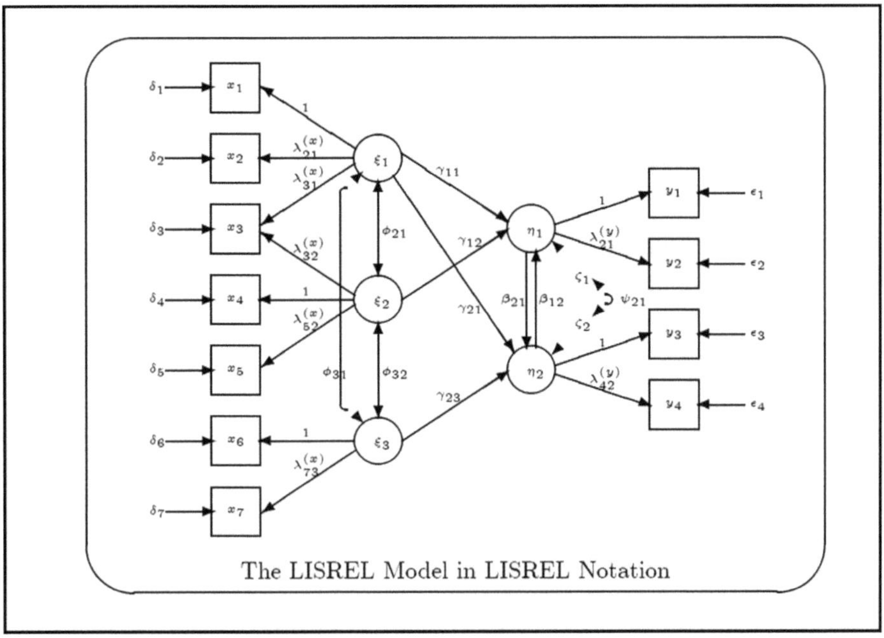

Fig. 2.5 Structural equation models with the LISREL model (Joreskog, 2007, p. 66). *Note* See Joreskog (2007) for a description of standard LISREL notation used for variables and arrows used in the model

science research. In their critique of common practices in applying SEMs, Bollen and Pearl (2013) note that "measurement issues are often given short shrift where the dimensionality of measures and appropriateness of indicators are not always discussed" (p. 324). Recent advances in SEMs include adding item response theory models within this approach. For example, bifactor models have been used to measure food insecurity (Tanaka et al., 2020). Also, various approaches using Rasch models have a similar structure to SEM approaches (Gochyyev & Wilson, 2018).

There are several important implications of SEM for this book. First of all, the use of diagrams to aid our conceptualization of the variables and their relationships to one another is important for guiding our thinking about Rasch measurement. Explanatory Rasch models are fundamentally about structural relationships. Next, some of the challenges posed by considering measurement issues in SEM based on factor analysis can be examined in detail with explanatory Rasch models. Finally, issues related to causality and SEM also appear in explanatory Rasch models and need to be carefully considered. In this book, explanatory Rasch models offer another approach for examining invariant structural relationships with a strong grounding in Rasch measurement theory.

Explanatory Item Response Models

> It is evident that the two approaches, the descriptive measurement approach and the explanatory approach, can be combined. Thus, explanation is seen as complementary to measurement. (De Boeck & Wilson, 2004, p. 3)

Explanatory item response models (EIRM) are a major focus of this book. De Boeck and Wilson (2004) edited an influential volume that summarized much of the previous work on these measurement models. A key feature of EIRMs is the addition of item and person covariates to item response models for measurement. The introduction of covariates for both items and persons provides the opportunity to examine structural relationships that can support explanatory analyses. Another key feature of EIRMs is that parameter estimation can be approached using generalized linear mixed models (McCulloch, 2003). The use of GLMMs opens up a host of options for linking measurement and explanation in the human sciences. EIRMs have been developed for a variety of item response models including the Rasch model (De Boeck & Wilson, 2004).

EIRMs include several key ideas. These are the distinction between descriptive and explanatory models, the use of fixed and random effects, estimation of model parameters with GLLMs, and graphical displays. EIRMs, as with other structural approaches, can be represented in graphical displays.

First of all, an important distinction can be made between descriptive and explanatory variables in EIRMs. EIRMs provide the opportunity to include item and person covariates as predictors in the model to create explanatory models. There are four general models that can be based on whether item and person predictors are included. The four models are called doubly descriptive, person explanatory, item explanatory, and doubly explanatory. Doubly descriptive models do not include any covariates, item explanatory models include item covariates, person explanatory models include person covariates, and doubly explanatory models include both item and person covariates. Each of these models are described in more detail later in the book.

A second important distinction that arises with EIRMs is the introduction of fixed and random effects into our conceptualization of measurement models. Fixed effects are parameter estimates that are constant in the model, while random effects are parameter estimates that are modeled to have a distribution (e.g., normal distribution). We will discuss the distinction between fixed and random effects further in Chap. 3. There are four Rasch models that can be identified based on various combinations of fixed and random effects (De Boeck, 2008). These four Rasch models are (1) the fixed persons—fixed items Rasch model (FPFI Rasch), (2) the random persons—fixed items Rasch model (RPFI Rasch), (3) the fixed persons—random items Rasch model (FPRI Rasch), and (4) the random person—random item Rasch model (RPRI Rasch). These Rasch models are interesting from both theoretical and model-data fit perspectives.

A third important feature of EIRMs is that the parameters in the models can be estimated with generalized linear mixed models (De Boeck & Wilson, 2004, 2016;

McCulloch, 2003). This statistical framework can be used for estimating the parameters of the descriptive Rasch models including the Dichotomous Model (Chap. 5), and Polytomous Models (Chap. 6).

A fourth feature of EIRMs is that they can be displayed graphically. Figure 2.6 illustrates the general form of the Rasch model from this perspective. There are three parts of GLLMs shown in this display. The first part is the random component that connects Y_{pi} and π_{pi} through a distribution function with π_{pi} representing the probability of person p responding positively to item i (Panel A). The next part is the link function that connects π_{pi} to η_{pi} using a logistic link (Panel B). The third part is the linear component that connects η_{pi} (logits) to two covariates or predictors (β_k and θ_{pj}) through design matrices X and Z (Panel C). The dotted circles indicate random effects, while the solid circles indicate fixed effects. Figure 2.7 shows the following models discussed in this book using the same type of graphical displays: Linear Logistic Rasch Model (Panel A), Latent Regression Rasch Model (Panel B), and Combined Covariates Rasch Model (Panel C).

In summary, all of the approaches within the structural tradition can be used to explore relationships between variables. Models in the structural tradition provide an approach for exploring causal relationships including the ideas about explanation and invariance as described by Woodward (2000). EIRMs are distinct from the other structural approaches in this section because they examine individual cases instead of focusing on reproducing covariances and correlations between variables. EIRMs

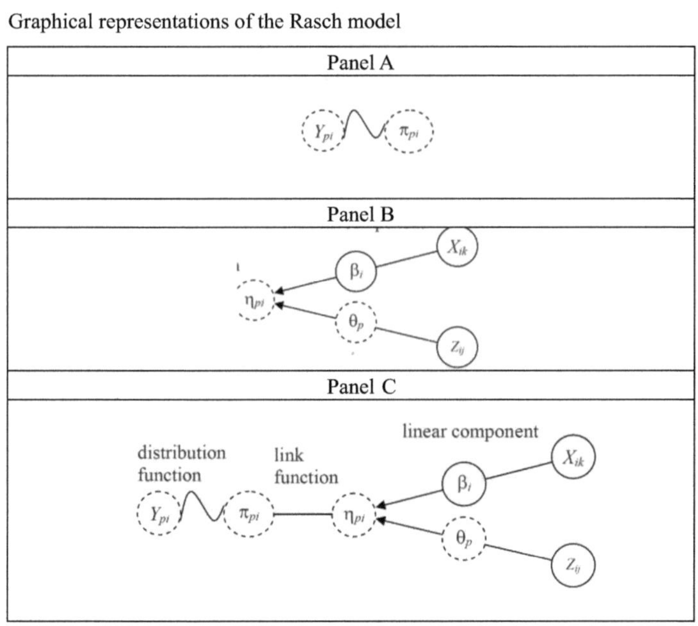

Fig. 2.6 Graphical representations of the Rasch model. *Note* Adapted from wilson et al. (2008, p. 92)

Graphical representation for three explanatory Rasch models

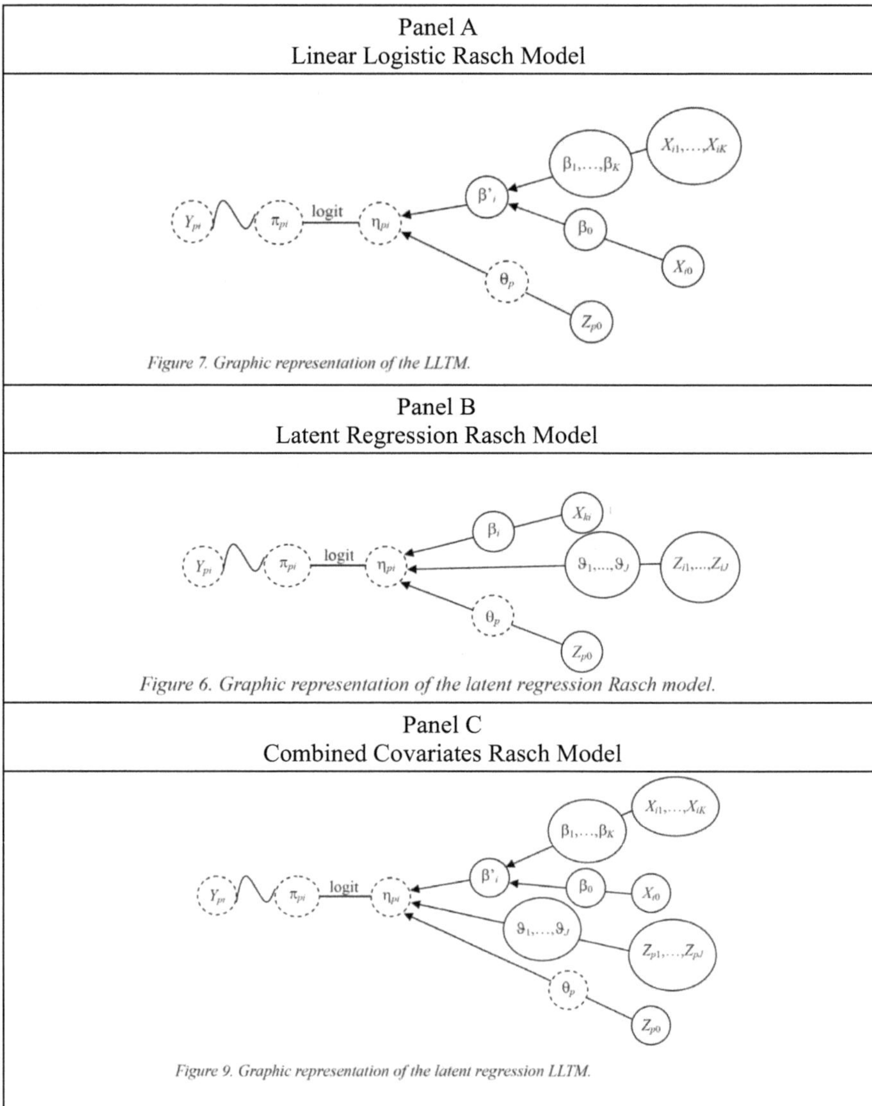

Fig. 2.7 Graphical representation for three explanatory Rasch models. *Note* Dotted circle indicates random variable, Beta is fixed item effect, Z is random design effect, X is fixed design effect, and theta is random person effect. See text within the chapter for a deeper description

can be used to provide explanations of the influences of various covariates (items, persons) on the probability of a positive response for each person. Evaluation of the quality of measurement can also be based on structural features of the measurement process (Maul et al., 2017).

Explanatory Rasch models are the focus of this book. As pointed out by Rost (2001), the extension of Rasch measurement theory to extended Rasch models is not direct. For example, the issue of unidimensionality is discussed in this section, but some explanatory Rasch models are inherently multidimensional. An important question to consider is the extent to which general principles of invariant measurement generalize to invariant structural relationships, as well as explanatory Rasch models.

In the next section, we highlight the use of Rasch measurement theory within the structural tradition. Explanatory Rasch models have the potential to guide the creation of invariant structural frameworks that supports both description and explanation with well-defined variables. Ideally, these well-defined variables reflect an invariant continuum as described earlier.

Guiding Principles for Measurement and Structural Analysis

The lessons from the previous two sections on measurement and explanation and invariance are summarized in this section. The guiding principles linking measurement and structural analyses are all based on invariance: The concept of invariance is the glue that binds everything together. Invariance has implications for both measurement processes and structural analyses that can guide our thinking about research and practice in the human sciences.

Summary of Invariance and Measurement

Table 2.5 summarizes the major principles that characterize our selected measurement theorists (Guttman, Lazarsfeld, Mokken, and Rasch). The summary is organized around four principles related to the construct, person measurement, item calibration, and structural analysis.

In terms of principles related to the construct, all four measurement theorists shared the idea that a construct can be defined by a unidimensional latent variable. Their perspectives on item-invariant person measurement are also remarkably similar, although they vary in the metric of the person scores obtained by different models. With the exception of Rasch, none of our selected measurement theorists explicitly discussed person response functions. The goals of person-invariant calibration of items (location of items on the continuum used to define the construct) was shared by Guttman, Lazarsfeld, and Rasch, while Mokken proposed the MH model that relaxes this aspect as an assumption. Item response functions (IRFs) were used

Table 2.5 Invariance and measurement

Principles	Guttman	Lazarsfeld	Mokken	Rasch
I. Construct				
Latent variable	Yes	Yes	Yes	Yes
Dimensionality	Unidimensional	Unidimensional	Unidimensional	Unidimensional
II. Person measurement				
Item-invariant measurement	Yes	Yes	MHM: Yes DMM: Yes	Yes
Person response functions	No	No	No	Yes
III. Item calibration				
Person-invariant calibration	Yes	Yes	MHM: No DMM: Yes	Yes
Item response functions	No	Yes	Yes	Yes
IV. Structural Aspects				
Items	Universe of items	Interchangeability of items		Comparisons
Persons	Populations		Explanatory relationships	Specific objectivity

Note Monotone homogeneity model (MHM; monotonically non-decreasing IRFs), Double Monotonicity Model (DMM; monotonically increasing and nonintersecting IRFs)

by all of the measurement theorists. Guttman did not explicitly create IRFs, but as shown in Fig. 2.2 (Panel A) an implicit step-like item response function can be used to represent Guttman scaling.

Even though the focus of their measurement theories was not specifically on issues related to explanatory models, each of our selected theorists has discussed several structural aspects of measurement. The combination of principles of invariant measurement and invariant relationships is a major theme of this book. The selected measurement theorists were primarily concerned with the creation of unidimensional scales, and yet there were adumbrations of issues related to invariant structural analyses within their work. For example, Guttman discussed the idea of populations, and this has implications for considering structural aspects of measurement models. Lazarsfeld's concept of interchangeability is another example that implies outside variables can and should be included in our considerations for developing scales. Mokken also considers structural aspects of measurement. In his words,

> It was the lack of any clear-cut explanatory relation of the data to the variable to be measured that inspired the search for other techniques by means of which the observations might be linked explicitly to a postulated, underlying variable in such a way that they would be open to empirical confirmation. After sufficient empirical verification of the appropriateness of the postulated relations, the underlying, explanatory variable might then be measured in terms of the inference provided by observations. (Mokken, 1971, p. 2)

Rasch also points out that "specific objectivity is not an absolute concept, and it is related to the specified frame of reference" (Rasch, 1977, p. 81). Specifically, he stresses that "systematic investigations are often structured as such interactions between two factors with all other factors of possible influence kept constant" (p. 81). Rasch's concept of specific objectivity can also be viewed as considering structural characteristics related to the conditions under which invariance is achieved. As pointed out by Andrich (2018), Rasch's perspective on invariant comparisons includes consideration of a specified frame of reference. These potentially objective comparisons extend measurement to include a consideration of the characteristics of the frame of reference that yields specific objectivity. One can argue that invariant comparisons within a frame of reference define scientific inquiry more generally. Andrich (2018) noted that it is possible for measurement models to go beyond description and to move toward explanations of person responses: "A measurement theory needs to not only merely describe the above properties of measurement, but also go to some length toward explaining them" (p. 71).

Summary of Explanation and Invariance

Turning now to explanation and invariance, the major principles underlying the four approaches (path analysis, factor analysis, structural equation modeling, and explanatory item response models) are summarized in Table 2.6. This summary is organized around four principles: Constructs, persons, items, and structural aspects. Each of these models can be considered in terms of how constructs are conceptualized.

A construct is a latent variable that can be viewed as having unidimensional, as well as multidimensional characteristics depending on the purpose of the measurements. A unidimensional construct can be conceptualized as a continuum with item and person locations on the latent variable. On the other hand, a multidimensional construct can be viewed as having several distinct domains that combine to define a single construct on this continuum. These domains are frequently observed in test blueprints and tables of specifications (Lane et al., 2016). For example, academic achievement may consist of quantitative and verbal domains that combine to form a unidimensional construct. For other purposes, academic achievement may be defined as a multidimensional construct with the quantitative and verbal domains being viewed separately. In this case, scores on assessments may be reported with both total and subtest scores. As with other measurement issues, an agreed-upon perspective on the targeted construct emerges over time within a community of scholars. The balance between these two views of dimensionality can be confusing in practice, and it has sometimes been called the "curse of dimensionality" (Bellman, 1957). For example, the curse of dimensionality within data mining refers to data sets with too many features. Multidimensional item response theory focuses on locating a person based on their responses within a common coordinate system that uses the same latent space across items and persons (Reckase, 2009). The underlying domains can be measured separately and used to define different subsets of items that define domain scores. These separate domain scores can be reported separately or combined in different ways to create an overall value for the underlying construct.

Table 2.6 Explanation and invariance

Principles	Path Analysis	Factor Analysis	Structural Equation Models	Explanatory Response Models
I. Constructs				
Multivariate	Yes	Yes	Yes	Yes
Multidimensional	No	Yes	Yes	Yes
Latent variables	No	Yes	Yes	Yes
Observed variables	Yes	No	Yes	Yes
Measurement model	Classical test theory	Factor analysis	Factor analysis	Rasch models
II. Persons				
Person scores	No	Sometimes	No	Between item dimensionality (subtests)
Path diagram	Yes	Yes	Yes	Yes
III. Items				
Item characteristics	No	Sometimes	Sometimes	Yes
Person and item displays				Variable map
IV. Structural Aspects				
Focus	Correlations between observed variables	Identify latent variables to account for observed correlations	Combine path and factor analyses	Model person responses
Multiple groups	Replications	Factorial invariance	Factorial invariance	Differential item functioning (measurement invariance)
Item covariates	No	No	Sometimes	Yes Linear logistic Rasch model (prediction of item difficulty)
Person covariates	Yes	No	Yes	Yes Latent regression Rasch model (prediction of person responses to items)
Invariant relationships	Causal analyses	Explanatory and confirmatory models	Explanatory and confirmatory models	Combined covariates Rasch model (item and person covariates)

Note Correlations or covariances can be used for these approaches. Multidimensional item response theory, Invariant structural relationships

It is also important to define how the term multivariate is used in this book. Multivariate statistics are typically defined by models that include multiple dependent variables. The goal is to explain the relationships between these dependent variables with other independent variables. Statistical analyses can be defined as being multivariate, while constructs are not defined in this way for the purposes of this book. Multivariate analyses are relevant for conceptualizing invariant structural relationships related to explanatory Rasch models. Although they start with a different focus from the measurement theorists, the implications of these approaches for explanation and invariance guide our perspectives on explanatory Rasch models.

In terms of the principles related to constructs (I. Constructs in Table 2.6), they are all multivariate in the sense defined above—there are multiple dependent and independent variables that are evaluated with the goal of finding invariant relationships. Path analysis as typically implemented does not focus on dimensionality or the use of latent variables. The other three approaches all use latent variables in analyses. Observed variables are included in all of the models with the exception of factor analysis that has the goal of identifying underlying latent variables or factors. The measurement model underlying path analysis is Classical Test Theory, while factor analysis is a measurement model that is used with structural equation models. In this book, Rasch measurement theory is used with explanatory response models.

The principles related to persons (II. Persons in Table 2.6) vary across approaches. Since these approaches are focusing on relationships between variables, person scores are not generally estimated for path analysis, factor analysis, and structural equation models. Because of their genesis in measurement models, explanatory response models frequently estimate person scores. Path diagrams can be used to illustrate the connections between variables in all of the approaches.

Turning now to items (III. Items in Table 2.6), item characteristics are not formally included in path analysis. Factor analysis and structural equation models can be used to examine item characteristics under some conditions (Reckase, 2009). Item characteristics are an explicit focus for explanatory response models.

Finally, structural aspects are the raison d'être for these approaches (IV. Structural aspects in Table 2.6). Path analysis, factor analysis, and structural equation models focus on reproducing the correlation or covariance matrices based on a set of simplifying conditions designed to summarize the matrices with fewer latent variables. Explanatory response models focus on modeling item-person responses by the addition of item and person covariates. A common way to examine invariance across multiple groups is to estimate the models using different subsets of persons. All of the models can use this simple strategy of replication or re-sampling to evaluate the stability and invariance of relationships. Factor analysis and structural equation modeling include the concept of factorial invariance to organize conceptualizing these analyses across groups, while differential item functioning (measurement invariance) is usually used with explanatory item response models. Person covariates are included in all of the approaches with the exception of factor analysis. Item covariates are featured with explanatory response models. Invariant relationships can be explored with all of the approaches shown in Table 2.6.

Discussion and Summary

> My focus on invariance is motivated by the claim that we-ordinary people and scientists alike-value invariant relationships... and that they are justified in doing so. (Woodward, 2021, p. 227)

This chapter examined perspectives on measurement, explanation, and invariance. All of the measurement theorists included here have carefully considered different facets of invariant measurement. They each had distinct views, but they all identified the goal of developing an invariant continuum that could be used to define a construct using a latent variable. The structural approaches discussed here were selected to connect principles of invariance across both measurement and structural analyses. The integration of ideas related to invariance, measurement, and explanation is a major theme of this book. This integration has important implications for progress in measurement and research in the human sciences.

A major goal of measurement is the creation of an invariant continuum for locating both items and persons on a line that can be used to represent a latent variable. Once we have calibrated scales to represent key constructs, then these scales can be used to discover invariant structural relationships among these variables. The structural framework provides a theory-based guide for explaining relationships among latent variables.

Figure 2.8 presents the relationships between the principles for invariant measurement and invariant relationships. The diagram indicates how invariance, measurement, and explanation fit together. We emphasize invariant scales in conjunction with invariant relationships. Invariance is the guiding principle for measurement and explanation. This framework guides the overall structure of the themes addressed in this book.

It is important to note that some researchers consider invariance to be a "siren's call" in psychometrics. Asún et al. (2017) worry that scientists delude themselves into believing that item response models are unconditionally invariant. We agree with their perspective that:

> the history of science shows that long-term results arise after having clear knowledge of the limitations of measurement tools, and not as a consequence of self-delusion about their properties. Believing that IRT models are methodological tools that yield internally and externally invariant measurement results means surrendering to the beauty of the sirens' call, but just as Ulysses tied himself firmly to the mast we must resist the call for the sake of our disciplines, by employing our best critical practices. (p. 403)

A similar comment can be made about the quest for invariant structural relationships. This chapter has described principles and best critical practices that can be used to guide research in thinking about both internal invariance (e.g., psychometric analyses) and external invariance (e.g., statistical analyses) as described by Asún et al. (2017).

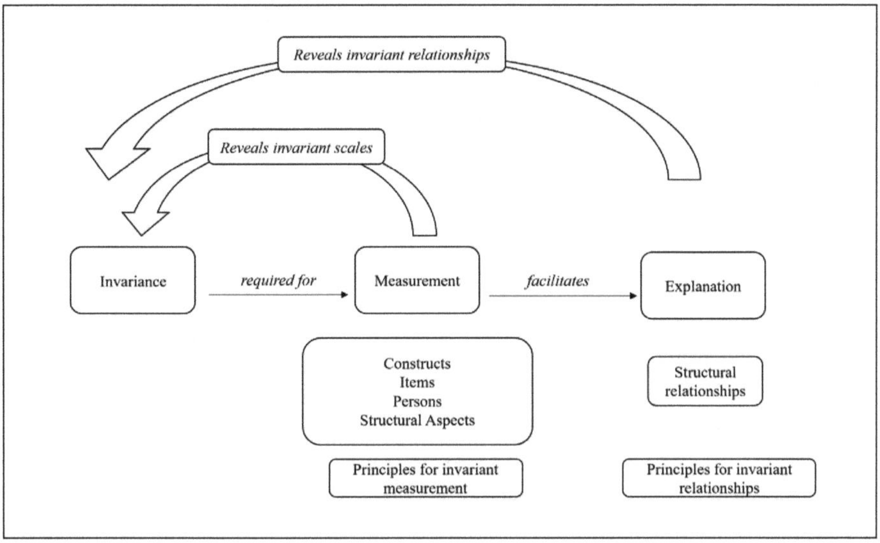

Fig. 2.8 Connections between invariance, measurement, and explanation

The principles discussed in this chapter have strong historical roots in measurement. Explanatory Rasch models provide an approach for conceptualizing issues related to measurement, invariance, and explanation. The principles discussed can also be viewed as requirements underlying an ideal-type perspective—in practice, model-data fit is essential for examining the correspondence between theory and the practical use of measurement models in the human sciences. Chapter 4 continues the topics discussed in chapter by examining specific strategies that can be used for examining model-data fit.

It should be stressed that one of the challenges in developing explanatory Rasch measurement theory is how to conceptualize the requirements of invariant relationships including well-developed scales based on Rasch measurement theory. It is important to note that model-data fit, including the specification of the limits on objectivity, is a key feature of explanatory measurement models. Both of these ideas are related to structural characteristics, and the potential limits on invariance that can be systematically explored and evaluated with suitable indices of model-data fit. A major goal of this book is to provide a careful consideration of invariance and its implications for measurement, as well as the examination of invariant relationships in structural models. We stress the extension of these scientific principles based on invariance to explanatory Rasch models. In particular, explanatory Rasch models include the opportunity to explore and define principles of invariance related to different frames of reference. Domains of invariance can be explained with a careful consideration of both item and person covariates in explanatory Rasch models.

In summary, the two main goals of this chapter were to integrate ideas related to invariant measurement and invariant structural relationships. The first goal of measurement is to create an invariant continuum for locating items and persons on a line to represent a latent variable. The second goal of explanation is to create an invariant structural framework to examine relationships between variables. As pointed by Simon (1990), "The fundamental goal of science is to find invariants" (p. 1).

References

Andrich, D. (1985). An elaboration of Guttman scaling with Rasch models for measurement. In N. B. Tuma (Ed.), *Sociological methodology* (pp. 33–80). Jossey-Bass.
Andrich, D. (2002). Understanding resistance to the data-model relationship in Rasch's paradigm: A reflection for the next generation. *Journal of Applied Measurement, 3*(3), 325–359.
Andrich, D. (2018). A Rasch measurement theory. In F. Guillemin et al. (Eds.), *Perceived health and adaptation in chronic disease* (pp. 66–91). Routledge.
Asún, R. A., Rdz-Navarro, K., & Alvarado, J. M. (2017). The sirens' call in psychometrics: The invariance of IRT models. *Theory & Psychology, 27*(3), 389–406.
Baker, F. B., & Kim, S. (2004). *Item response theory: Parameter estimation techniques. Second edition, revised and expanded*. Marcel Dekker.
Bartholomew, D. J. (2007). Three faces of factor analysis. In R. Cudeck & R. C. MacCallum (Eds.), *Factor analysis at 100: Historical developments and future directions* (pp. 9–21). Lawrence Erlbaum Associates Publishers.
Bellman, R. (1957). *Dynamic programming*. Princeton University Press.
Bollen, K. A. (1989). *Structural equations with latent variables*. John Wiley & Sons.
Bollen, K. A., & Pearl, J. (2013). Eight myths about causality and structural equation models. In S. Morgan (Ed.), *Handbook of causal analysis for social research. Handbooks of sociology and social research*. Springer.
Bond, T., Yan, Z., & Heene, M. (2020). *Applying the Rasch model: Fundamental measurement in the human sciences*. Routledge.
Cattell, J. M. (1893). Mental measurement. *The Philosophical Review, 2*(3), 316–332.
Cudeck, R., & MacCallum, R. C. (Eds.). (2007). *Factor analysis at 100: Historical developments and future directions*. Routledge.
De Boeck, P. (2008). Random item IRT models. *Psychometrika, 73*, 533–559.
De Boeck, P., & Wilson, M. (2004). *Explanatory item response models: A generalized linear and nonlinear approach*. Springer.
De Boeck, P., & Wilson, M. R. (2016). (Eds.). Explanatory response models. In W. J. van der Linden (Ed.), *Handbook of item response theory, volume one* (pp. 593–608). Chapman and Hall/CRC.
Duncan, O. D. (1966). Path analysis: Sociological examples. *American Journal of Sociology, 72*, 1–16.
Engelhard, G. (1984). Thorndike, Thurstone and Rasch: A comparison of their methods of scaling psychological and educational tests. *Applied Psychological Measurement, 8*, 21–38.
Engelhard, G. (1991). Thorndike, Thurstone and Rasch: A comparison of their approaches to item-invariant measurement. *Journal of Research and Development in Education, 24*(2), 45–60.
Engelhard, G. (1992). Historical views of invariance: Evidence from the measurement theories of Thorndike, Thurstone and Rasch. *Educational and Psychological Measurement, 52*(2), 275–292.
Engelhard, G. (1994). Historical views of the concept of invariance in measurement theory. In M. Wilson (Ed.), *Objective measurement: Theory into practice* (Vol. 2, pp. 73–99). Ablex.
Engelhard, G. (2005). Guttman scaling. In K. Kempf-Leonard (Ed.), *Encyclopedia of social measurement* (Vol. 2., pp. 167–174). Academic.
Engelhard, G. (2013). *Invariant measurement: Using Rasch models in the social, behavioral, and health sciences*. Routledge.

Engelhard, G., & Wang, J. (2024). *Invariant measurement: Using Rasch models in the social, behavioral, and health sciences* (2nd ed.). Routledge.
Gochyyev, P., & Wilson, M. (2018). Hierarchical and higher-order factor structures in the Rasch tradition: A didactic. *Journal of Applied Measurement, 19*(4), 338–362.
Godfrey-Smith, P. (2003). *Theory and reality: An introduction to the philosophy of science.* The University of Chicago Press.
Gould, S. J. (1996). *Mismeasure of man.* WW Norton & company.
Guttman, L. (1944). A basis for scaling qualitative data. *American Sociological Review, 9*(2), 139–150.
Guttman, L. (1950). The basis for scalogram analysis. In S. A. Stouffer, L. Guttman, E. A. Suchman, P. F. Lazarsfeld, S. A. Star, & J. A. Clausen (Eds.), *Measurement and prediction* (Vol. IV, pp. 60–90). Princeton University Press.
Holland, P. W., & Wainer, H. (Eds.). (1993). *Differential item functioning.* Psychology Press.
Joreskog, K. G. (1966). Testing a simple structure hypothesis in factor analysis. *Psychometrika, 31*, 165–178.
Joreskog, K. G. (1969). A general approach to confirmatory maximum likelihood factor analysis. *Psychometrika, 34*, 183–202.
Joreskog, K. G. (2007). Factor analysis and its extensions. In R. Cudeck & R. C. MacCallum (Eds.), *Factor analysis at 100: Historical developments and future directions* (pp. 47–77). Lawrence Erlbaum Associates Publishers.
Kuhn, T. S. (1970). *The structure of scientific revolutions* (2nd ed.). Princeton University Press.
Lane, S., Raymond, M. R., & Haladyna, T. M. (Eds.). (2016). *Handbook of test development.* Routledge.
Lawley, D. N., & Maxwell, A. E. (1971). *Factor analysis as a statistical method* (2nd ed.). Butterworth.
Lazarsfeld, P. (1966). Concept formation and measurement in the behavioral sciences: Some historical observations. In G. J. Direnzo (Ed.), *Concepts, theory, and explanation in the behavioral sciences* (pp. 144–202). Random House.
Lazarsfeld, P. (1968). Measurement. In T. Parsons (Ed.), *American sociology: Perspectives, problems, methods* (pp. 93–106). Basic Books, Inc.
Lazarsfeld, P. F. (1950a). The logical and mathematical foundation of latent structure analysis. In S. A. Stouffer, L. Guttman, E. A. Suchman, P. F. Lazarsfeld, S. A. Star, & J. A. Clausen (Eds.), *Measurement and prediction* (pp. 362–412). Princeton University of Press.
Lazarsfeld, P. F. (1950b). The interpretation and computation of some latent structures. In S. A. Stouffer, L. Guttman, E. A. Suchman, P. F. Lazarsfeld, S. A. Star, & J. A. Clausen (Eds.), *Measurement and prediction* (pp. 413–472). Princeton University of Press.
Lazarsfeld, P. F. (1958). Evidence and inference in social research. In D. Lerner (Ed.), *Evidence and inference* (pp. 107–138). The Free Press.
Lazarsfeld, P. F. (1959). Latent structure analysis. In S. Koch (Ed.), *Psychology: A study of a science* (*Formulation of the person and the social context*) (Vol. 3, pp. 476–543). McGraw-Hill.
Lazarsfeld, P. F. (1960). Latent structure analysis and test theory. In H. Gulliksen & S. Messick (Eds.), *Psychological scaling* (pp. 83–95). Wiley.
Lazarsfeld, P. F., & Henry, N. W. (1968). *Latent structure analysis.* Houghton-Mifflin.
Mari, L., Wilson, M., & Maul, A. (2021). *Measurement across the sciences.* Springer.
Meredith, W. (1993). Measurement invariance, factor analysis and factorial invariance. *Psychometrika, 58*, 525–543.
Millsap, R. E. (2011). *Statistical approaches to measurement invariance.* Routledge.
Mokken, R. J. (1971). A theory and procedure of scale analysis. In *The Hague.* De Gruyter.
Mokken, R. J. (1997). Nonparametric models for dichotomous responses. In W. J. van der Linden & R. K. Hambleton (Eds.), *Handbook of modern item response theory* (pp. 351–367). Springer.
Mokken, R. J., & Lewis, C. (1982). A nonparametric approach to the analysis of dichotomous item responses. *Applied Psychological Measurement, 6*, 417–430.

Mulaik, S. A. (1986). Factor analysis and Psychometrika: Major developments. *Psychometrika, 51*, 23–33.
Nozick, R. (1998). Invariance and objectivity. *Proceedings and Addresses of the American Philosophical Association, 72*(2), 21–48.
Nozick, R. (2001). *Invariances: The structure of the objective world*. Harvard University Press.
Pastor, D. A., & Finney, S. J. (2015). Promoting the use of path diagrams in quantitative research. In M. McCrudden, G. Schraw, & C. Buckendahl (Eds.), *Use of visual displays in research and testing: Coding, interpreting, and reporting data* (pp. 111–144). Information Age.
Pearl, J. (2018). *The book of why*. Basic Books.
Rasch. (1960/1980). *Probabilistic models for some intelligence and attainment tests* (Expanded edition, Chicago: University of Chicago Press, 1980). Danish Institute for Educational Research.
Rasch, G. (1961). On general laws and meaning of measurement in psychology. In J. Neyman (Ed.), *Proceedings of the fourth Berkeley symposium on mathematical statistics and probability* (pp. 321–333). University of California Press.
Rasch, G. (1977). On specific objectivity: An attempt at formalizing the request for generality and validity of scientific statements. *Danish Yearbook of Philosophy, 14*, 58–94.
Reckase, M. D. (2009). *Multidimensional item response theory*. Springer.
Rost, J. (2001). The growing family of Rasch models. In A. Boomsa, M. A. J. van Duijn, & T. A. B. Snijders (Eds.), *Essays on item response theory* (pp. 25–42). Springer.
Sijtsma, K., & Molenaar, I. W. (2016). Mokken models. In W. J. van der Linden (Ed.), *Handbook of item response theory: Volume 1: Models* (pp. 303–321). CRC press.
Spearman, C. (1904). General intelligence objectively determined and measured. *American Journal of Psychology, 15*, 201–293.
Stevens, S. S. (1946). On the theory of scales of measurement. *Science, 103*(2684), 677–680.
Tanaka, V., Engelhard, G., & Rabbitt, M. P. (2020). Using a Bifactor model to measure food insecurity in households with children. *Journal of Family and Economic Issues, 41*(3), 492–504.
Thorndike, E. L. (1904). *An introduction to the theory of mental and social measurements*. Teachers College, Columbia University.
Thurstone, L. L. (1931). *The reliability and validity of tests*. Edwards.
Thurstone, L. L. (1935). *The vectors of mind*. University of Chicago Press.
Thurstone, L. L. (1947). *Multiple factor analysis*. University of Chicago Press.
Wind, S. A. (2017). An instructional module on Mokken scale analysis. *Educational Measurement: Issues and Practice, 36*(2), 50–66.
Woodward, J. (2000). Explanation and invariance in the special sciences. *The British Journal for the Philosophy of Science, 51*(2), 197–254.
Woodward, J. (2021). *Causation with a human face: Normative theory and descriptive psychology*. Oxford University Press.
Wright, S. (1921). Correlation and causation. *Journal of Agricultural Research, 20*, 557–585.
Wright, S. (1934). The method of path coefficients. *The Annals of Mathematical Statistics, 5*(3), 161–215.
Yule, G. U. (1912). On the methods of measuring association between two attributes. *Journal of the Royal Statistical Society, 49*(6), 579–652.

Chapter 3
Rasch Measurement Theory and Generalized Linear Mixed Models

> *Our thesis is that a common core of statistical models [and] item response models [can be] framed within the broad family of GLMMs* (De Boeck & Wilson, 2004, p. 38)

The purpose of this chapter is to describe in broad strokes the underlying statistical aspects of generalized linear mixed models. Rasch models (Rasch, 1960/1980) can be productively viewed through the lens of generalized linear mixed models. The extensions of the Rasch family of models discussed in this book are based on generalized linear mixed models. These models provide a solid statistical grounding for the extended Rasch models discussed in this book.

This chapter is organized as follows. The first section includes a brief description of the relationships between linear regression models, generalized linear models, mixed models, and generalized linear mixed models. Next, we show how a generalized linear mixed model can be used to estimate the parameters of the dichotomous Rasch model. Finally, we illustrate how a generalized linear mixed model can be used to estimate the dichotomous Rasch model for the Learning Stimulation Scale introduced in Chap. 1.

What Are Generalized Linear Mixed Models?

In order to answer this question, this section provides a brief description of the relationships between linear regression models, generalized linear models, linear mixed models, and generalized linear mixed models. The treatment here is brief given the purposes of this book. For more details regarding these models, we recommend that readers refer to McCulloch et al. (2008).

G. Engelhard and S. A. Wind, *Invariant Measurement with Explanatory Rasch Models in the Human Sciences*, https://doi.org/10.1007/978-3-032-08816-1_3

Linear Regression Model

There is a long history of linear models in statistics that goes back to Gauss and Legendre, who developed these models in astronomy (Stigler, 1981). For example, linear models were developed to represent the relationship between the positions of planets and stars based on the observations of astronomers. It was widely recognized that these observations varied based on potential measurement errors that varied across astronomers. A detailed consideration of these error distributions led to the concept of a Gaussian or Normal distribution of errors, and to the quest for methods to minimize the effects of these errors (McCullagh & Nelder, 1983). Reflecting this goal, the simple linear regression model is a linear model that predicts a dependent variable (Y) using values of an independent variable (X) with an error term (ε).

The linear regression model can be written as

$$Y_i = \beta_0 + \beta_1 X_i + \varepsilon_i \tag{3.1}$$

where the term $\beta_0 + \beta_1 X_i$ is defined as the mean response when $X = X_i$. The residuals (ε_i) are assumed to be independent and normally distributed with a mean of 0 and variance of σ^2. The parameters in the model are β_0 (intercept), β_1 (slope), and σ^2 (variance). This model represents a straight-line plot with Y_i as a continuous dependent variable and X_i as the independent variable.

Figure 3.1 (Panel A) shows a linear relationship between X (e.g., level of achievement) and a continuous dependent variable Y_1 (e.g., test scores) with no residual error ($\varepsilon_i = 0$). The illustrative data used to construct this model are shown in Table 3.1

A basic linear model is illustrated in Fig. 3.2 (Panel A). The units for both independent and dependent variables are logits. The equation for this model is

$$\hat{Y}_i = 0.747 + 1.093_1 X_i$$

The intercept (0.747) is shown with a horizontal line that indicates the point where X is zero. The slope of the line is 1.093, which indicates that an increase of one unit in X leads to an increase of 1.093 units in Y. $\hat{Y}_i$ is the expected value based on the model. In the next section, these parameters are interpreted in terms of the generalized linear model with dichotomous data within the context of measurement.

In many cases, the dependent variable of interest is not continuous. Figure 3.1 (Panel B) illustrates a dichotomous dependent variable (Y = 0, 1) predicted by a continuous independent variable. This plot is not very useful for drawing inferences about the relationship between the two variables because the dependent variable is limited to two categories. One approach to analyzing dichotomous responses is to group the independent variable into meaningful categories, and then count the number of events (Y = 1) in each category. Then, the relationship between values of the independent variable and the count of observations can be plotted and interpreted. The development of this approach was an important advance in the history of linear models with the extension of linear models to categorical data, such as the counts of

Table 3.1 Illustrative data for 10 persons

	Independent variable	Dependent variables					
Person	X	Y_1	Y_2	Y_3	Y_4	Y_5	$\hat{Y}_6$
1	−4.00	5	0	0.02	−4.00	−3.17	−3.62
2	−3.00	10	0	0.05	−3.00	−3.28	−2.53
3	−2.00	15	0	0.12	−2.00	−2.36	−1.44
4	−1.00	20	0	0.27	−1.00	−0.91	−0.35
5	0.00	25	1	0.50	0.00	2.25	0.75
6	1.00	30	1	0.73	1.00	1.83	1.84
7	2.00	35	1	0.88	2.00	3.31	2.93
8	3.00	40	1	0.95	3.00	5.50	4.03
9	4.00	45	1	0.98	4.00	5.17	5.12
10	5.00	50	1	0.99	5.00	4.57	6.21

Note X = independent variable (e.g., level of achievement), Y_1 = continuous dependent variable (e.g., test score), Y_2 = dichotomous dependent variable (e.g., responses to a test item), Y_3 = probabilities as dependent variable (e.g., probability of correct responses to a test item at each score level), Y_4 = logistic transformation of probabilities (e.g., log odds of probabilities of correct responses), Y_5= Y_4 with random normal error (Mean = 0, SD = 1), and $\hat{Y}_6$ = expected value based on linear model.

events. A classic example of this approach is Bortkewitsch's (1898) analysis of the count of the number of soldiers kicked to death by Prussian horses. Fig. 3.1 (Panel C) shows the probabilities of events grouped into categories (e.g., test score ranges) for an independent variable. As illustrated in Fig. 3.1 Panel C, the use of probabilities to define the dependent variable tends to yield non-linear relationships.

Generalized Linear Model

The next major conceptual breakthrough for analyzing categorical data was the development of generalized linear models using the tools developed for linear models (Azen & Walker, 2011; McCullagh & Nelder, 1983). The key idea underlying generalized linear models is that a transformation of a categorical dependent variable (Y) is more likely than an untransformed Y to yield a linear relationship with an independent variable (X). The transformation is important because it provides the opportunity to utilize the machinery developed for analyzing linear models. There are several transformations of proportions that are commonly used to achieve a linear relationship. Some common transformations are Binomial, Gaussian, Gamma, and Poisson. These are described in detail in Azen and Walker (2011). The Binomial transformation is used here because the logistic distribution has close connections to the Rasch model.

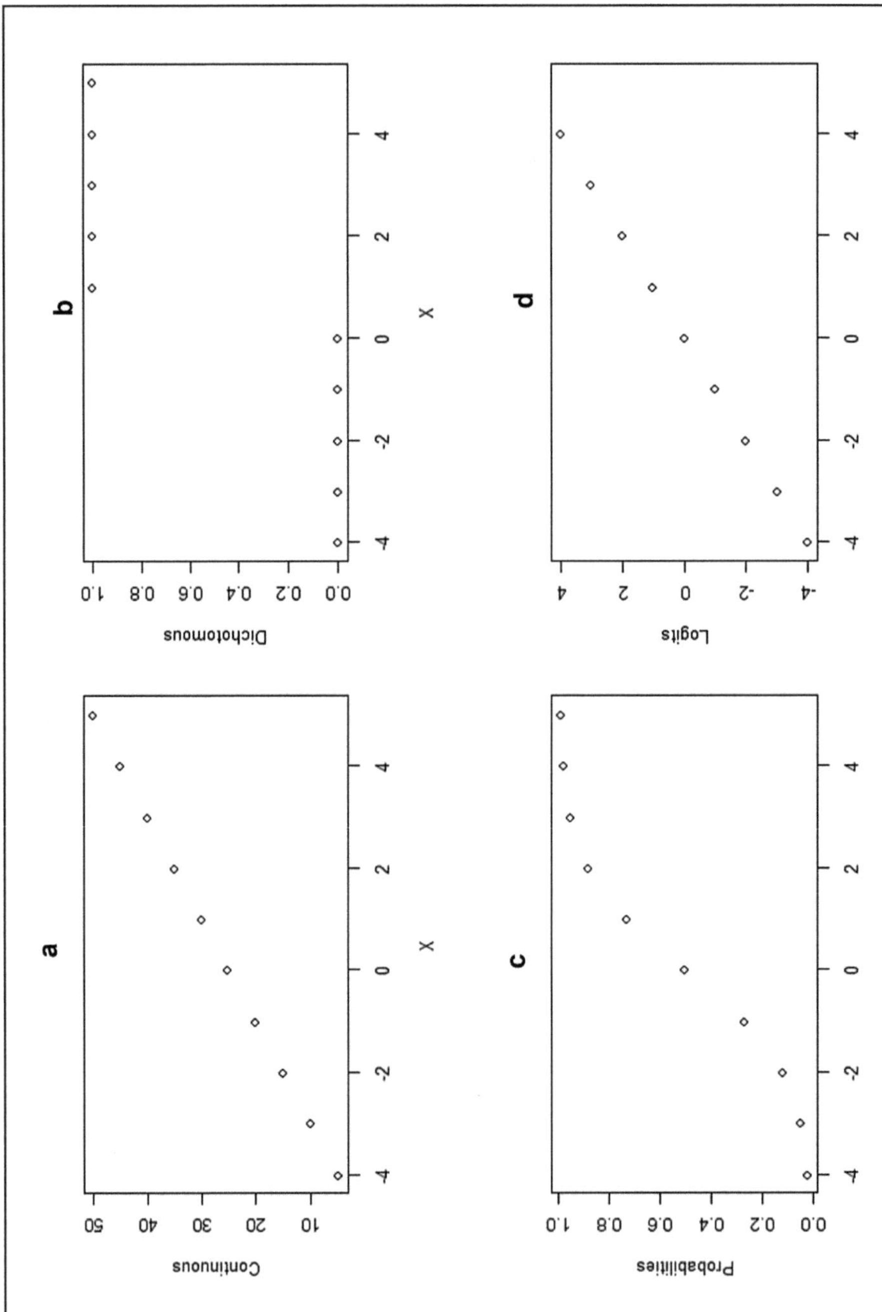

Fig. 3.1 Scatterplots for illustrative data with different dependent variables

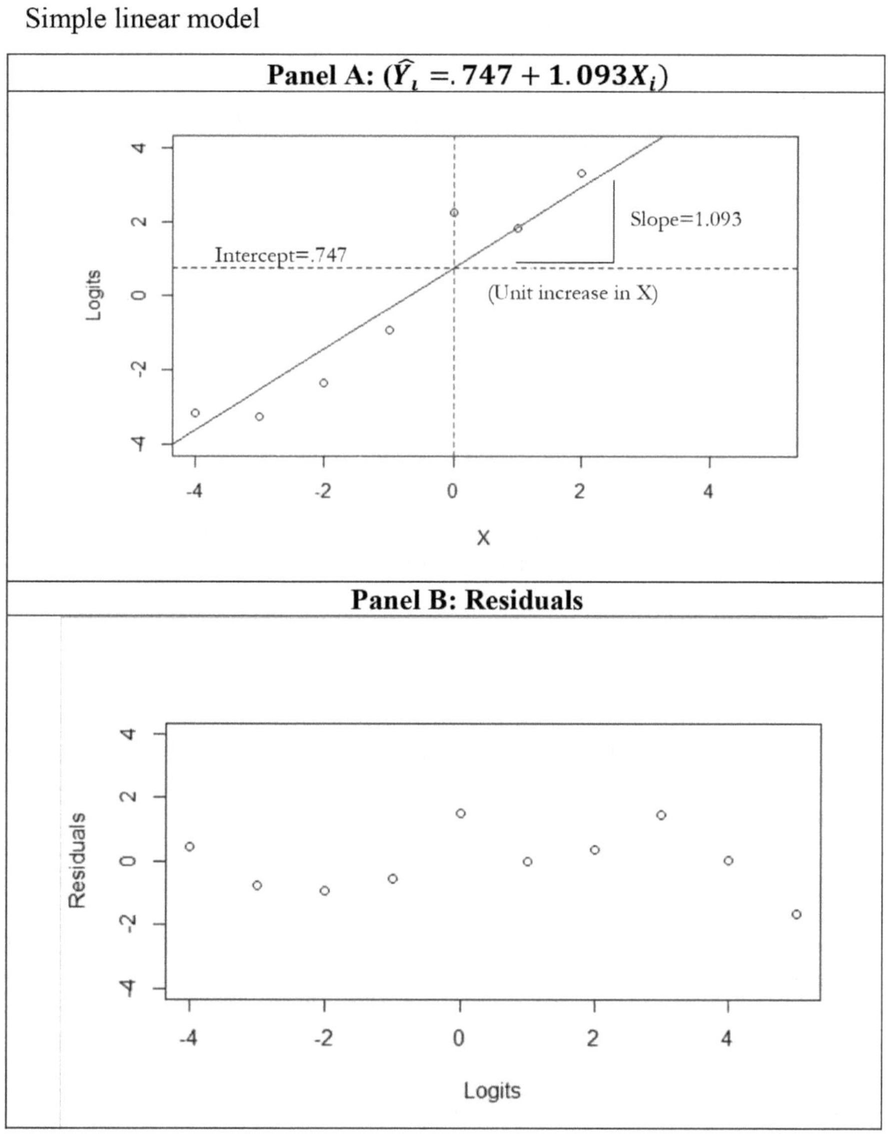

Fig. 3.2 Simple linear model

A generalized linear model for predicting a dichotomous outcome can also be written in a similar fashion. First, we can express the probability for a response in category 1 of the dichotomous outcome variable (Y = 1) using the exponential form:

$$\Pr(Y = 1|X) = \pi(X) = \frac{\exp(\beta_0 + \beta_1 X_i)}{1 + \exp(\beta_0 + \beta_1 X_i)} \tag{3.2}$$

where $Pr(Y = 1|X)$ is the conditional probability $\pi(X)$ of observing Y = 1 given X.

The parameters in the model have a comparable meaning to those in the simple linear regression model presented earlier with β_0 as the intercept and β_1 as the slope. These parameters can also be incorporated into an exponential form, and this can be written using a logistic transformation:

$$g(X) = \ln(\pi(X)/(1 - (\pi(X)) \tag{3.3}$$

where $g(X)$ are logits, and $\pi(X)$ is the conditional probability of observing Y = 1 given X. This can also be expressed as a linear model:

$$g(X) = \beta_0 + \beta_1 X_i \tag{3.4}$$

where g(.) is a link function (logit function for Rasch models).

Figure 3.1 (Panel D) shows the linear relationship obtained after the logistic transformation of the probabilities from Table 3.1. Figure 3.2 (Panel A) shows the relationship between X and Y_4 with a random error component with e ~ N(0, 1). The residual plot is shown in Fig. 3.2 (Panel B) (Table 3.2)

Linear Mixed Model

Linear mixed models include both fixed and random effects. These models were designed to address data with a group structure such as nested models and hierarchical models. For example, the structure of schooling includes an inherent nested structure with students nested within classrooms that are nested within schools and districts. This nested structure introduces a variety of issues that cannot be appropriately modeled using simple linear regression models.

Mixed models explicitly recognize that grouped data are common in many applications (Faraway 2016). Grouped data includes observations with a hierarchical or nested structure, and mixed models provide a framework for examining this structure.

The combination of generalized linear models and mixed models is called generalized linear mixed models. These models provide a very powerful statistical framework for estimating a variety of Rasch models.

Generalized Linear Mixed Models

Generalized linear mixed models (GLMMs) reflect an important extension to generalized linear models. By definition, GLMMs include both fixed and random effects. As pointed out earlier, fixed effects are levels of a covariate that are considered unknown constant parameters to be estimated in a linear model. Random effects are levels of a covariate that are modeled as a random sample from a distribution.

Table 3.2 Person by item matrix for learning stimulation scale (40 persons, 11 items)

Person	Education level	Items										
		1	2	3	4	5	6	7	8	9	10	11
1	3	1	1	1	1	1	1	1	1	1	1	1
2	2	1	0	0	1	0	1	1	1	1	0	1
3	2	1	1	0	1	1	1	1	1	0	0	1
4	2	1	0	1	1	1	1	1	1	0	1	1
5	2	1	0	1	1	1	0	1	0	0	1	1
6	3	1	1	0	1	1	1	1	1	1	1	1
7	1	1	1	0	1	0	0	0	0	0	0	0
8	3	1	1	1	1	1	1	1	0	1	1	1
9	3	1	1	1	1	1	1	1	1	1	1	1
10	2	1	0	0	1	1	1	0	1	1	0	1
11	2	1	1	0	1	0	1	1	1	0	0	1
12	2	1	0	0	1	1	1	1	1	0	0	1
13	1	1	0	1	1	0	1	0	1	0	0	1
14	1	1	0	1	1	0	1	0	1	0	0	1
15	2	1	1	1	1	1	1	1	1	0	0	1
16	1	1	0	0	1	0	1	0	0	1	0	1
17	1	1	0	0	1	1	1	1	0	0	0	1
18	2	1	1	0	1	0	1	1	0	1	0	1
19	1	0	0	0	0	0	1	0	0	0	0	1
20	1	1	0	0	1	0	1	0	1	0	0	1
21	1	1	0	0	1	1	0	0	0	0	0	1
22	2	0	0	1	1	0	1	1	1	1	0	1
23	2	1	0	1	1	1	0	1	1	0	1	1
24	1	0	0	1	1	1	0	0	1	1	0	1
25	2	1	1	0	1	1	1	1	1	0	1	1
26	1	0	0	0	0	0	0	1	0	1	0	1
27	3	1	1	1	1	1	1	1	1	0	1	1
28	3	1	1	1	1	1	1	1	1	1	1	1
29	3	1	1	1	1	1	1	1	1	0	0	1
30	2	1	1	0	1	0	1	1	0	1	0	1
31	3	1	1	0	1	1	1	1	1	1	0	1
32	1	1	0	0	1	1	1	1	0	0	0	1
33	1	0	0	0	1	0	0	0	0	0	0	1
34	3	1	1	0	1	1	1	1	1	1	1	1

(continued)

Table 3.2 (continued)

Person	Education level	Items										
		1	2	3	4	5	6	7	8	9	10	11
35	1	1	0	0	1	0	1	0	1	0	1	1
36	1	1	0	0	0	0	1	0	0	0	0	0
37	1	1	1	0	1	1	1	0	0	0	0	1
38	2	1	0	0	1	1	1	1	0	0	1	1
39	3	1	1	1	1	1	1	1	1	1	0	1
40	2	1	1	0	1	0	1	1	1	1	0	1

Note Cell entries indicate that the items are present (x = 1) or not present (x = 0) for 40 homes. Education level represents an estimate of mother's education (1 = Low, 2 = Medium, 3 = High) based on additional information

GLMMs can be viewed as an extension of the generalized linear model (McCulloch et al., 2008) with both fixed and random effects. The inclusion of random effects provides the potential for a wide range of models for analyzing grouped data (Azen & Walker, 2011; McCullagh & Nelder, 1983). GLMMs can be written as

$$g(.) = \theta Z - \beta X \tag{3.5}$$

where g(.) is the logit link function. The first part of the right side of the equation reflects random effects, where Z is a design matrix and θ reflects one or more random effects. Next, X is a design matrix, and β reflects fixed effects. A detailed description of GLMMs is provided in McCulloch et al. (2008).

GLMMs play a key role in estimating the parameters for the family of descriptive Rasch models and the extensions to explanatory Rasch models. In the next section, we discuss the use of GLMMs for estimating the dichotomous Rasch model.

Estimating the Dichotomous Model with a Generalized Linear Mixed Model

The parameters of the Dichotomous Model can be estimated by using the generalized linear mixed model (GLMM) framework described in the previous section. The probability of a positive response from person *n* on item *i* based on the Dichotomous Model can be written as

$$\pi_{ni1} = \frac{\exp(\theta_n - \delta_i)}{1 + \exp(\theta_n - \delta_i)} \tag{3.6}$$

where θ_n is the location of person *n*, and δ_i is the location of item *i* on the latent variable. These probabilities can be transformed into logit form as

$$\eta_{ni} = \ln\left[\frac{\pi_{ni1}}{1 - \pi_{ni1}}\right] = \theta_n - \delta_i \tag{3.7}$$

with the same definitions of the parameters as Eq. 3.6.

If we assume that a person's response to an item ($X_{ni} = 1$) is drawn from a binomial distribution with a probability of P_{ni} (X_{ni})~$binomial(1, P_{ni})$, then we can write the Dichotomous Model in GLMM format as

$$\eta_{ni} = \theta_0 - \delta_1 X_i \tag{3.8}$$

In this case, θ_0 is a random person effect (intercept), while δ_1 is the fixed item effect or location of an item on the latent variable, and X_i is an item design effect. This view of θ_0 as a random effect also underlies marginal maximum likelihood estimation that is widely used to estimate the parameters of item response theory models (Baker & Kim, 2004).

Illustration

The Learning Stimulation Scale from Chap. 1 is used in this section to illustrate the estimation of the Dichotomous Model with a GLMM. We use the EIRM package for R (Bulut, 2021) throughout this book to estimate a variety of Rasch models based on GLMMs. The EIRM package is a wrapper around the lme4 package (Bates, 2010; Bates & Sarkar, 2007). The EIRM package provides the basic tools for estimating several Rasch models, including the creation of Wright maps.

Steps for Conducting GLMM Analyses

There are several steps for preparing the data and carrying out the GLMM analysis using the EIRM package. The major steps include:

- Data editing and preparation
    - Format data: Wide to long data format
    - Coding of covariates: items and persons
- Syntax (model specification):
    - Model statement
    - Fixed and random effects
- Interpretation:
    - Item locations
    - Wright Map

- Model-data fit:
  - Overall fit
  - Item fit
  - Person fit

The EIRM package does not include detailed model-data fit analyses as part of its standard functions. Model-data fit indices for Rasch models are discussed in Chap. 4. This additional model-data fit information includes summary tables for item, person, and overall fit, as well as several of the common indices that are reported as a routine part of Rasch analyses, such as reliability of item and person separation. A critical review of the model-data fit indices is essential for a complete interpretation and evaluation of the results. The desirable invariance properties of Rasch models are only realized when there is good model-data fit.

Learning Stimulation Scale

The first step is to re-shape the item response data to long format, which is required for the application of GLMMs. Item response data are typically stored in wide format, with each row representing a single person and item responses shown in columns. An example of wide-format person-by-item response data is shown in Table 3.3. One tool with which to create a long format for these data is the reshape2 package in R (Wickham, 2020). In our example, we used the melt() function from this package, which requires users to specify the variable used to identify cases (id.vars), variable names for the items (variable.name), and a label to be used for the responses after the data are re-shaped (value.name):

Table 3.3 Wide to long format (5 persons, 4 items)

Wide format

	Person	I1	I2	I3	I4
1	1	1	1	1	1
2	2	1	0	0	1
3	3	1	1	0	1
4	4	1	0	1	1
5	5	1	0	1	1

Long format

	Person	Item	Response
1	1	I1	1
2	2	I1	1
3	3	I1	1
4	4	I1	1
5	5	I1	1
6	1	I2	1
7	2	I2	0
8	3	I2	1
9	4	I2	0
10	5	I2	0
11	1	I3	1
12	2	I3	0
13	3	I3	0
14	4	I3	1
15	5	I3	1
16	1	I4	1
17	2	I4	1
18	3	I4	1
19	4	I4	1
20	5	I4	1

```
library(reshape2)
longdata <- melt(data, id.vars=c("Person"), variable.name =
"Item", value.name = "Response")
```

Table 3.3 shows the re-shaped data for 5 persons on the first 4 items created using this code. For the dichotomous Rasch model, there are no covariates to be coded. We will demonstrate the use of covariates in later chapters.

The next step is to create the syntax for analyzing the long-format data. The formula for specifying the Rasch model is quite simple in the EIRM package:

Response ~ -1+Item+(1|Person)

The response variable is dichotomous (0,1). The items are defined as a fixed effect (Item), and the persons are modeled as a random effect, which is specified using the number 1 and a pipe symbol (1|Person). The −1 value in the place of the intercept indicates that the model does not include an intercept. The EIRM package can be used to obtain the estimated parameters using the EIRM() function with the formula and data specified as follows:

```
library(EIRM)
Rasch <- EIRM(formula = "Response~-1+Item+(1|Person)", data
= longdata).
```

When the EIRM function is applied to the data, the Rasch model is estimated. We can interpret the results by examining the item locations and the Wright Map. This information can be obtained using the print() function to display the item difficulty parameters and the plot() function to display a Wright Map to illustrate the distributions of item and person parameters:

```
print(Rasch, difficulty = TRUE) # To get difficulty parameters
plot(Rasch,difficulty = TRUE) # Wright Map
```

By default, the EIRM() function calculates item easiness parameters. In order to obtain item difficulty parameters, it is necessary to specify "difficulty = TRUE" in both the print() and plot() function commands. The item locations are given in Table 3.4. The estimated item difficulties match the values shown in Table 1.4 in Chap. 1.

A Wright Map (labeled by default as "Person-Item Map") is shown in Fig. 3.3. It shows the item locations on the latent variable (Latent dimension). The easiest item is Item 11 (−3.76 logits), while the hardest item is Item 10 (1.01 logits). It should be noted that in these analyses that the item difficulties are not centered at zero, which is common practice in many Rasch analyses. The distribution of the persons is also

Table 3.4 Item calibrations for the learning stimulation scale

Item Number	EIRM calibration		
	Item location	SE	Standardized
1	−2.58	0.59	−0.93
2	0.14	0.42	0.73
3	0.71	0.43	1.08
4	−3.26	0.72	−1.34
5	−0.55	0.43	0.31
6	−2.08	0.53	−0.62
7	−1.00	0.45	0.04
8	−0.70	0.43	0.22
9	0.42	0.43	0.90
10	1.01	0.44	1.26
11	−3.76	0.85	−1.65
Mean	−1.06	0.52	0.00
SD	1.64	0.14	1.00

Note Item locations obtained used EIRM package with marginal maximum likelihood estimation. The item locations can be estimated as item difficulty as shown here or as item easiness

shown (labeled "Person parameter distribution") on the Wright Map. The person locations are centered at zero. The earlier Wright Map in Chap. 1 was created using the Facets Computer Program (Linacre, 1989). Appendix A shows the full R code for running the illustration.

Discussion and Summary

In summary, the purpose of this chapter was to provide a concise description of linear models, mixed models, generalized linear models, and generalized linear mixed models. GLMMs can be used to estimate the item and person parameters of the dichotomous Rasch model. The Learning Stimulation Scale from Chap. 1 are used to illustrate the estimation of the Rasch model using the EIRM package (Bulut, 2021).

The basic ideas in this chapter are expanded and illustrated in future chapters. Chapter 4 considers aspects of model-data fit related to the original family of Rasch models, and the extensions based on GLMMs. Chapter 5 continues the presentation of Rasch models for dichotomous data, and describes extensions to the model. Chapter 6 focuses on Rasch models for polytomous data. Chapter 7 extends these ideas to rater-mediated assessments.

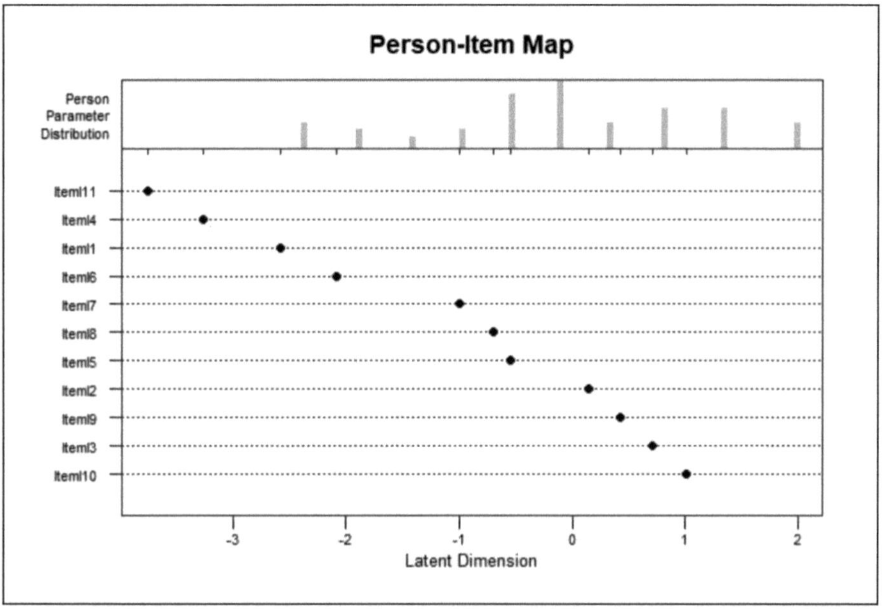

Fig. 3.3 Wright Map. *Note* This version of a Wright Map was obtained in R using the EIRM package (Bulut, 2021)

Appendix A: C3-Learning Stimulation Scale-Illustration.R

```
rm(list=ls(all=TRUE))
library(reshape2)
library(EIRM)

Location <- getwd()
setwd(Location)
data <- read.csv("HomeData_Original.csv", header = TRUE)
longdata <- melt(data, id.vars=c("Person"), variable.name =
"Item",
value.name = "Response")
Rasch <- EIRM(formula = "Response~-1+Item+(1|Person)", data =
longdata)
print(Rasch, difficulty = TRUE) # To get item difficulty
parameters

## EIRM formula: "Response~-1+Item+(1|Person)"
##
## Number of persons: 40
##
## Number of observations: 440
##
## Number of predictors: 11
##
## Parameter Estimates:
```

```
##
## Difficulty S.E. z-value p-value
## ItemI1 -2.5779722 0.5914585 4.3586699 1.308553e-05
## ItemI2 0.1436178 0.4221002 -0.3402457 7.336715e-01
## ItemI3 0.7074812 0.4318813 -1.6381379 1.013929e-01
## ItemI4 -3.2614148 0.7194289 4.5333385 5.805867e-06
## ItemI5 -0.5526148 0.4292869 1.2872855 1.979948e-01
## ItemI6 -2.0788059 0.5271728 3.9433099 8.036471e-05
## ItemI7 -0.9962854 0.4451887 2.2378948 2.522792e-02
## ItemI8 -0.6968731 0.4334557 1.6077147 1.078977e-01
## ItemI9 0.4218840 0.4251417 -0.9923374 3.210330e-01
## ItemI10 1.0065542 0.4431022 -2.2716071 2.311025e-02
## ItemI11 -3.7573360 0.8524826 4.4075224 1.045598e-05
##
## Note: The estimated parameters above represent 'difficulty'.
```

```
plot(Rasch, difficulty = TRUE) # Wright Map
```

References

Azen, R., & Walker, C. M. (2011). *Categorical data analysis for the behavioral and social sciences.* Routledge.

Baker, F. B., & Kim, S. (2004). *Item response theory: Parameter estimation techniques* (Second edition, Revised and expanded ed.). Marcel Dekker.

Bates, D., & Sarkar, D. (2007). *lme4: Linear Mixed-Effects Models Using S4 Classes.* R package version 0.9975–12.

Bates, D. M. (2010). *lme4: Mixed-effects modeling with R.* Retrieved from http://lme4.r-forge.r-project.org/book/

Bortkewitsch, L. V. (1898). *Das gesetz der kleinen zahlen.* Teubner.

Bulut, O. (2021). *EIRM: Explanatory item response modeling for dichotomous and polytomous item responses* [Computer software]. Retrieved from http://CRAN.R-project.org/package=EIRM.

De Boeck, P., & Wilson, M. (Eds.). (2004). *Explanatory item response models: A generalized linear and nonlinear approach.* Springer.

Faraway, J. J. (2016). *Extending the linear model with R: Generalized linear, mixed effects and nonparametric regression models.* Chapman and Hall/CRC.

Linacre, J. M. (1989). *Many-facet Rasch measurement.* MESA Press.

McCullagh, P., & Nelder, J. A. (1983). *Generalized Linear Models.* Chapman Hall.

McCulloch, C. E., Searle, S. R., & Neuhaus, J. M. (2008). *Generalized, linear, and mixed models.* John Wiley & Sons, Inc.

Rasch. (1960/1980). *Probabilistic models for some intelligence and attainment tests* (Expanded edition, Chicago: University of Chicago Press, 1980). Danish Institute for Educational Research.

Stigler, S. M. (1981). Gauss and the invention of least squares. *The Annals of Statistics*, 465–474.

Wickham, H. (2020). *Reshape2: Flexibly Reshape Data: A Reboot of the Reshape Package* [WWW Document]. URL https://cran.r-project.org/package=reshape2.

Chapter 4
Evaluating Measurement Quality for Dichotomous Rasch Models

Models should not be true, but it is important that they are applicable

(Rasch, 1960/1980, pp. 37-38)

Researchers use a variety of techniques to evaluate statistical and psychometric models to ensure that the results from these models can be meaningfully interpreted and used. For example, diagnostic tests of fit are used to evaluate assumptions for linear regression models. These assumptions include examining the following questions: (1) Are residuals are normally distributed? (2) Are residuals statistically independent from one another? and (3) Do the residuals exhibit homoscedasticity? These tests of fit are often conducted as part of the model diagnostics that help researchers evaluate and compare the applicability of linear regression models (Wasserman, 2010).

Rasch measurement theory approaches the evaluation of measurement quality in a way that is distinct from traditional model-data fit analyses in statistics and other popular IRT models, such as the two-and three-parameter logistic models (Baker & Kim, 2004). Rasch measurement theory evaluates measurement quality based on the idea that the model reflects fundamental measurement properties to which measurement data must adhere in order to yield desirable properties related to invariant measurement.

Researchers using a Rasch-based approach begin their analyses with a model, and then evaluate their data for evidence that item response patterns match the guiding principles that undergird the model. Rasch measurement theory can be viewed as developing models with specific conditions and principles defined relative to invariance broadly conceived. In other approaches to measurement, researchers apply several candidate models to their data, and then compare the model-data fit results to identify a model that best reflects the characteristics of the data. This philosophical difference in approach to model-data fit is an important theoretical distinction between Rasch measurement theory and other measurement traditions.

G. Engelhard and S. A. Wind, *Invariant Measurement with Explanatory Rasch Models in the Human Sciences*, https://doi.org/10.1007/978-3-032-08816-1_4

It should be stressed that residual analyses play an important role in all of the methods used to evaluate model-data fit for Rasch models. Residual-based statistics reflect discrepancies between model-based predicted and observed responses. Residuals are useful for evaluating model-data fit because they allow researchers to begin with the hypothesis that their data adhere to the principles of Rasch measurement theory, and then explore deviations from those requirements to inform next steps. Residuals are one of the pillars of statistics identified by (Stigler, 2016), as well as a foundational pillar of measurement wisdom (Engelhard, 2022).

In this chapter, we focus on methods for evaluating the measurement quality of Rasch measurement analyses that include various approaches to evaluating model-data fit. We use the dichotomous Rasch model as the basis for our illustrations before considering model-data fit for polytomous and extended models. The remainder of the chapter is organized as follows. First, we start with a discussion of model-data fit. As we will show, many indicators of model-data fit for Rasch models are based on detailed analyses of residuals. Next, aspects of model-data fit are presented with a focus on three aspects: Construct focus, item focus, and person focus. This section presents several methods that can be used to evaluate the principles of invariant measurement for Rasch models. The following section illustrates these model-data fit indices using the Learning Stimulation Scale that was introduced in Chap. 1.

Model-Data Fit

There are numerous indices that can be used to evaluate the psychometric quality of Rasch models. This section focuses on three general aspects that are commonly used in the literature on Rasch measurement theory. We group these aspects into three general categories based on the focus of the indicators: construct focus, item focus, and person focus. Table 4.1 provides an overview of these three general aspects of model-data fit including the underlying questions and methods related to each aspect. These aspects are described in the following sections.

Construct Focus

A key aspect of evaluating measurement quality is the theoretical conceptualization and empirical representation of the construct or latent variable. It is helpful to consider four questions related to the construct measured by the scale:

- Do the locations of the items and persons on the variable map reflect the expected locations?
- Does the Wright Map make sense based on previous research and theory on construct?
- How well does a single construct explain variation in person responses?

Table 4.1 Aspects of model-data fit

	Aspects	Questions	Methods
1.0	Construct focus		
1.1	Variable map	Do the locations of the items and persons on the variable map reflect the expected locations? Does the variable map make sense based on previous research and theory on construct?	Graphical representation of construct
1.2	Unidimensionality	How well does a single construct explain variation in person responses? Are item responses associated with additional constructs beyond what can be explained by the primary construct?	Percent of variance explained by model Inter-item correlations of residuals Local independence (Q3 statistic) Principal components analysis of residuals
1.3	Overall model-data fit	How well does the model fit overall? Which model provides the best model-data fit (model-comparison)?	Information criteria: AIC, BIC, Deviance Comparison of models (baseline, Rasch)
1.4	General structural aspects	What are the key predictors for item and person locations on the construct?	Variable map with covariates
2.0	Item focus		
2.1	Item locations	Is the item hierarchy reasonable?	Theoretical justification
2.2	Item fit	Are individual items associated with unexpected responses? Are the item response functions monotonically increasing on the latent variable?	Infit/Outfit MSE Fit categories (A, B, C, D) Item response functions (graphical displays)
2.3	Item separation on latent variable	Are item locations spread out on the latent variable?	Reliability of item separation index
2.4	Structural aspects: Item covariates	How well do the item classifications predict item locations?	Linear logistic Rasch Model Locations of item classifications Comparison of fit
3.0	Person focus		
3.1	Person locations	Are the person locations reasonable?	Theoretical justification

(continued)

Table 4.1 (continued)

	Aspects	Questions	Methods
3.2	Person fit	Are persons associated with unexpected responses? Are person response functions monotonically decreasing on the latent variable?	Infit/Outfit MSE Fit categories (A, B, C, D) Person response functions (graphical displays)
3.3	Person separation on latent variable	Are person locations spread out on the latent variable?	Reliability of person separation index
3.4	Structural aspects: Person covariates	How well do person categories predict person locations?	Latent regression Rasch model Locations of person categories Comparison of fit

- Are item responses associated with additional constructs beyond what can be explained by the primary construct?
- How well does the model fit overall?

The answers to these questions provide inter-related evidence for the adequacy of the representation of the construct.

Variable Map

At their core, measurement theories provide a theoretical framework for defining a construct and latent variable. The conceptualization and development of a useful scale is the *sin qua non* of measurement. In Rasch measurement theory, variable maps provide a graphical representation of the construct. The dichotomous Rasch model provides the simplest example of how to use item and person locations to define a line as a variable map. The variable map is sometimes called an item map, construct map, and Wright map.

The variable map is a visual representation of the latent variable. It shows the location of both persons and items on an underlying continuum or line. An example of a variable map was shown in Fig. 1.1 in Chap. 1. The variable map provides a display that can be used to provide support regarding the meaningfulness of the item order, as well as the location of persons the latent variable. Important questions regarding the interpretation of the variable map include:

- Do the locations of items and persons match expected locations?
- Does the variable map make sense based on previous research and theory on construct?

Unidimensionality

The first principle of Rasch measurement theory specifies the necessity of creation of a unidimensional scale to represent a construct. Key questions related to evaluating unidimensionality include:

- How well does a single construct explain variation in person responses?
- Are item responses associated with additional constructs beyond what can be explained by the primary construct?

Several sources of evidence can be used to evaluate the unidimensionality of a set of items created to represent the construct, including:

- Percent of variance explained by model
- Inter-item correlations of residuals
- Local independence (Q3 statistic)
- Principal components analysis of residuals

Each of these approaches is based on the analysis of residuals.

In conducting residual analyses to evaluate model-data fit, the first step is to apply the selected Rasch model to the data to obtain parameter estimates for item and person locations. These parameter estimates are then used to calculate expected responses for each item-person combination. Model-expected responses are subtracted from these observed responses to calculate residuals. Residuals (Y_{ni}) are calculated for each item-person combination as:

$$Y_{ni} = X_{ni} - E_{ni}, \tag{4.1}$$

where X_{ni} is person n's response to item i, and E_{ni} is the response that would be expected given person and item location estimates from the model. Positive residuals indicate that the observed response was higher than expected, and negative residuals indicate that the observed response was lower than expected. To avoid cancelation effects associated with combining positive and negative residuals, these values can be transformed to standardized residuals (Z_{ni}) as follows:

$$Z_{ni} = Y_{ni}/\sqrt{W_{ni}}, \tag{4.2}$$

where W_{ni} is the variance of the observed response (X_{ni}):

$$W_{ni} = \sum_{k=0}^{M_i} (k - E_{ni})^2 p_{nik}, \tag{4.3}$$

where p_{nik} is the probability for a response in Category k from test-taker n on item i, and M_i is the maximum score for item i. Figure 4.1 provides an illustration of this definition of residuals.

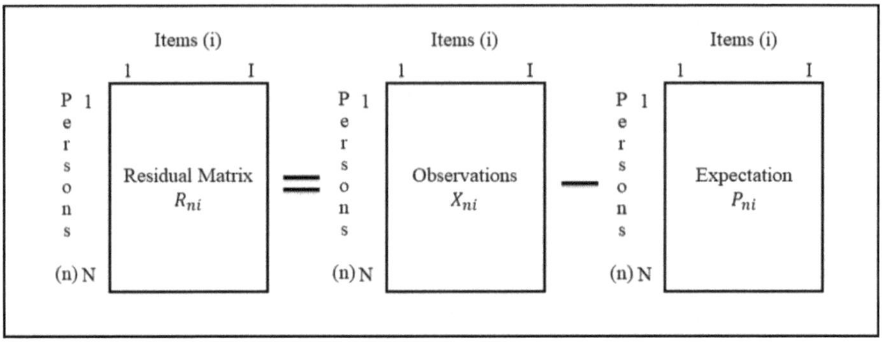

Fig. 4.1 Definition of residuals

These residuals can be used to estimate the percent of variance explained by the model. Higher estimates of explained variance provide support for unidimensionality. Following Linacre (2003), we can calculate the proportion of variance in the responses associated with the Rasch model estimates as

$$\text{Proportion of Explained Variance} = [\text{Var(Observed)} - \text{Var(Residuals)}]/\text{Var(Observed)}$$

where Var(Observed) = variance of the observations, and Var(Residuals) is the variance of the residuals. This provides an estimate of the proportion of variance in item responses that can be explained by the Rasch model. Many researchers use a critical value of 20% of variance explained by Rasch measures as evidence of adequate adherence to unidimensionality to support the interpretation of Rasch model results for many practical purposes (Reckase, 1979). Please see Linacre (2003) for more details and considerations on this topic.

In addition to examining the proportion of explained variance, correlations between the residuals can be calculated and examined. The underlying motivation for examining the residual correlations is to detect additional structure between the items after controlling for the unidimensional construct.

These residual correlations can be used for another model-data fit procedure that evaluates local independence. The local independence principle states that item responses should be independent after controlling for the construct or latent variable. In other words, the construct should explain the relationships between person responses to different items. Adherence to local independence is important because it implies that location estimates for individual items can be interpreted independently from the other items in the analysis. In other words, any associations between item responses should be a result of the primary latent variable. Violations of local independence can occur for a variety of reasons, including multidimensionality or construct-irrelevant item characteristics, such as item response formats or overlapping content. When local independence is violated, estimates of person location parameters and reliability may be compromised (Marais, 2013).

Several methods are available for evaluating local independence. A popular technique for this purpose is to simply examine the magnitude of inter-item residual correlations. The idea behind this analysis is that if item responses are independent, the errors associated with individual items will not be related to any other items. In this case, small inter-item residual correlations provide evidence of adherence to local independence. Yen (1984) discussed this technique and proposed the Q3 statistic. Q3 is calculated for pairs of items as the Pearson correlation between residuals associated with each item.

If the local independence principle is met, Q3 statistics should be close to zero for all item pairs. Researchers have proposed various methods for determining critical values and upper limits for these statistics that indicate meaningful violations of local independence (Christensen et al., 2017). Results from methodological studies on Q3 suggest that single critical values cannot be universally applied across studies. Instead, researchers have recommended considering the overall distribution of Q3 for a given dataset and examining the relative magnitude of these statistics for individual item pairs relative to the average value (Marais, 2013). Reflecting this perspective, Christensen et al. (2017) conducted a simulation study to examine various approaches to evaluating values of Q3 for evidence of local independence violations. These researchers suggest values that exceed the average inter-item residual correlation by 0.2 or 0.3 may indicate potential or substantial violations of local independence, respectively. Researchers should interpret Q3 statistics as a tool for identifying pairs of items that may include dependent responses, and to consider these values in combination with other indicators of model-data fit. The expected value of Q3 is slightly smaller than zero under local independence, and an adjusted Q3 (aQ3) statistic obtained by subtracting the average Q3 is recommended for interpretation (Chen et al., 2013).

Principal components analysis (PCA) can also be used to explore whether or not additional patterns exist in the correlations between residuals. PCA of residuals (PCA-R) is also be used to evaluate the dimensionality of the data after fitting a Rasch model (Chou & Wang, 2010; Linacre, 1998). This technique is different from standalone PCA techniques as they are often used in general statistical applications. Rather than applying PCA directly to item responses, the PCA-R is applied to standardized residuals after a Rasch model is applied. The idea behind this approach is that Rasch model estimates reflect the primary latent variable that explains the item responses. If unidimensionality holds, then there should not be any meaningful patterns of relationships in the residuals.

Results from PCA-R of standardized residuals should not be interpreted using guidelines from typical standalone PCA or factor analysis because the procedures are based on different types of data and serve different purposes. In PCA-R of standardized residuals, eigenvalues reflect the magnitude of any patterns in the residuals that may reflect secondary latent variables. Accordingly, eigenvalues from PCA-R are called "contrasts" because they reflect potential contrasting latent variables from the primary latent variable. Researchers can evaluate the size of these contrasts to determine whether any potential secondary dimensions are small enough to suggest adequate adherence to unidimensionality.

Researchers have discussed several methods for identifying critical values to classify contrasts (eigenvalues) as evidence of adequate unidimensionality. Linacre (2020) suggests that eigenvalues less than about 2.00 suggest adequate unidimensionality for most purposes. Several other researchers used simulations and real-data analyses to explore various approaches to interpreting eigenvalues from standardized residual PCA. In general, these researchers do not recommend using a single critical value to evaluate eigenvalues for evidence of unidimensionality (Chou & Wang, 2010; Raiche, 2005; Wind & Schumacker, 2021) because these values are sensitive to many aspects of the analysis, including item and person sample sizes. On the other hand, Karabatsos (2000) criticized the use of this procedure in general, observing that standardized residuals may not be appropriately distributed for use with parametric statistical procedures such as PCA and that this procedure may underestimate misfit between the Rasch model and empirical data. Despite these criticisms, many researchers use this approach as part of their Rasch model analyses (Wind & Schumacker, 2021). In practice, researchers should consider standardized residual PCA as another tool for exploring the alignment between empirical data and requirement for unidimensionality underlying descriptive Rasch models. Results from PCA-R should be interpreted in combination with other indicators of model-data fit.

Overall Model-Data Fit

Overall model-data fit indices provide another source of evidence about how well a unidimensional model fits the data. In traditional Rasch analyses, overall model-data fit is not stressed; however, we suggest comparing the Rasch model to explanatory models as a baseline model. One reason for including this step is that it provides a framework for extending the model-data fit indices to explanatory Rasch models with item and person covariates that are used in future chapters in this book. The key questions are:

- How well does the model fit overall?
- Which model provides the best model-data fit (model-comparison)?

Overall model-data fit is typically examined using information statistics (Cohen & Cho, 2016). Commonly used indices include Akaike Information Criteria (AIC), Bayesian Information Criteria (BIC) statistics, and deviance statistics. These information criteria are based on adjustments to the log likelihood (LogL). AIC can be calculated by using $-2\text{logL} + 2q$ (Akaike, 1973), BIC can be calculated by using $-2\text{logL} + \text{q}\ln(N)$ (Schwarz, 1978), in which q is the number of parameters and N is the sample size. Deviance can be calculated by using -2LogL (McCullagh, 2019).

Information statistics can also be used to compare two or more candidate models during model selection (Vrieze, 2012). The main objective is to select the model that loses the least amount of information. In terms of the interpretation of these information criteria, a smaller number suggests a better model fit. In some applications, researchers can calculate likelihood ratio statistics, and compare these values between models using techniques such as chi-square tests or analysis of variance (ANOVA) models. For example, the *anova* function in R can be used to compare a baseline model with the Rasch model.

In summary, information criteria summarize the degree to which a given model can represent the characteristics of a set of data. These indices reflect the amount of information that is lost by using a particular model to represent a data set. Smaller values indicate that less information is lost, indicating better model fit. Researchers can evaluate AIC, BIC, and deviance statistics for several candidate models to identify the model with the smallest value that indicates better model-data fit. In our research, we have found it useful to compare the fit of the Rasch model to a baseline model. There are several candidates for baseline models that can be used depending on the context of the research.

General Structural Aspects

Although the dichotomous Rasch model discussed in this chapter does not include item or person covariates, model-data fit evaluation includes general structural aspects that begin to emerge when we consider the concept of specific objectivity (Rasch, 1977). The quest for objectivity includes a consideration of the conditions that yield invariance—it is important to examine explicitly whether or not invariance is achieved under a variety of conditions. Simply fitting the Rasch model is not enough to achieve invariance without detailed analyses of the specific circumstance where the models do or do not work with a particular data set. In future chapters, we discuss how these structural aspects play a role in the extended Rasch models that include item and person covariates.

Item Focus

Items play an essential role in evaluating measurement quality. It is important to consider both the content of the items, the location of the items on the variable map, and the theoretical justification for defining the construct using the items. It is helpful to consider five questions related to item results:

- Is the item hierarchy reasonable?
- Are individual items associated with unexpected responses?
- Are the item response functions monotonically increasing on the latent variable?
- Are item locations spread out on the latent variable?
- How well do the item classifications predict item locations?

The answers to these questions provide inter-related evidence for the adequacy of the item-based representation of the construct.

Item Locations

The variable map with item locations plays an important role in illustrating the meaning of a construct. In examining the variable map, the following question should be considered:

- Is the item hierarchy reasonable?

The item order is evaluated based on the empirical item locations, and also the theoretical justification that may explain the locations. These locations can also be modeled using explanatory Rasch models that provide additional insight into the underlying processes related to item characteristics that affect item locations. This information can be used as evidence related to construct validity.

Item Fit

Individual items can be evaluated for model-data fit. The two guiding questions for examining item fit are:

- Are individual items associated with unexpected responses?
- Are the empirical item response functions monotonically increasing on the latent variable?

Item fit can be evaluated using the following techniques:

- Infit/Outfit *MSE*
- Fit categories (A, B, C, D)
- Item response functions (graphical displays)

We discuss each of these techniques in the following paragraphs.

The first step in residual-based model-data fit analysis is to apply the selected Rasch model to the data to obtain parameter estimates for items and persons. These parameter estimates are then used to calculate expected responses for each item-person combination. Model-expected responses are subtracted from observed responses to calculate residuals as shown in Eq. 4.1. Positive residuals indicate that the observed response was higher than expected, and negative residuals indicate that the observed response was lower than expected. Standardized residuals can also be used to examine item fit as shown in Eqs. 4.2 and 4.3.

It is common practice in Rasch measurement applications to summarize residuals for individual elements using mean square error (*MSE*) statistics (Smith & Plackner, 2009). These statistics provide a numeric summary of the frequency and magnitude of residuals associated with individual elements. Researchers often use two *MSE* statistics in Rasch analyses. First, outfit *MSE* is an unweighted mean of standardized residuals associated with an element of a measurement procedure, such as an item or person. Because it is an unweighted mean, outfit *MSE* is sensitive to outliers. In a residual analysis context, outliers reflect large discrepancies between model-expected and observed responses. For example, in an achievement test, a large residual may occur if a student with a low location (i.e., low achievement) provided a correct response to a difficult item.

For example, in the Learning Stimulation Scale example from Chap. 1, a large residual may occur for an item if a home with a low overall level of stimulation had an item with a high level of stimulation. For items, outfit *MSE* is calculated as the unweighted average of the squared standardized residuals associated with responses to the item of interest:

$$\textit{Outfit MSE} = \sum_{n=1}^{N} Z_{ni}^2 / N, \tag{4.4}$$

where N is the number of observed responses to item i. Outfit *MSE* can also be calculated for persons as the average of the residuals for all of the responses associated with a person of interest.

Infit *MSE* statistics are an alternative residual summary statistic similar to outfit *MSE* that are weighted by response variance to reduce the impact of outliers. For items, infit *MSE* is calculated as:

$$\textit{Infit MSE} = \sum_{n=1}^{N} W_{ni} Z_{ni}^2 / \sum_{n=1}^{N} W_{ni}. \tag{4.5}$$

Like outfit *MSE*, infit *MSE* for persons is calculated as the weighted mean of residuals associated with a person of interest.

The Rasch measurement literature includes many discussions and recommendations related to the appropriate interpretation and use of *MSE* statistics (e.g., Karabatsos, 2000; Linacre & Wright, 1994; Seol, 2016; Smith, 2004; Wolfe, 2013; Wu & Adams, 2013). Researchers have proposed a variety of critical values and methods for evaluating fit statistics that reflect different measurement purposes, sample size considerations, response format considerations, among other characteristics. However, most researchers who have studied these statistics tend to agree on several properties of these statistics. First, values close to 1.00 generally indicate acceptable fit. Second, values lower than 1.00 indicate a less-variable response pattern than expected given parameter estimates. Less variation than expected could result from a variety of factors, such as dependencies between items or range restrictions in category use. Third, values greater than 1.00 indicate more variation in response patterns than expected given parameter estimates. Higher-than-expected *MSE* fit statistics often indicate haphazard response patterns (i.e., "noisy" responses) that are often more cause for concern than lower *MSE* fit statistics (Bond et al., 2020). It should be noted that standardized infit and outfit statistics are available; however, we do not use them in this book. Wright and Masters (1982) provides a description of how to calculate the standardized *MSE* statistic. Several R packages, including the TAM package, include options to obtain these standardized MSE statistics. Researchers can also calculate standardized residuals independent of package functions by applying Eqs. 4.1 through 4.3.

Researchers can interpret *MSE* statistics as continuous variables rather than focusing on classifying items, persons, or other elements as "fitting" or "misfitting," and use these statistics alongside other fit indicators to identify elements of a measurement procedure that may warrant additional consideration. However, it is also useful to summarize *MSE* statistics by categorizing fit categories using a framework proposed by Engelhard and Wind (2018) and Engelhard and Wang (2021): (A) productive for measurement ($0.50 \leq MSE \leq 1.50$); (B) less productive but not distorting measures ($MSE < 0.50$); (C) unproductive but not distorting measures ($1.50 \leq MSE < 2.00$); and (D) unproductive and distorting measures ($MSE > 2.00$). Of course, these values and interpretations can vary depending on the particular context of the measurement situation.

Empirical versions of item response functions can be visualized using graphical displays of residuals. These displays provide additional evidence for exploring model-data fit for Rasch models. Specifically, we can construct plots that illustrate residuals associated with items, persons, or other elements of interest. Several methods are available for visualizing Rasch model residuals. Another useful method for visualizing and exploring residuals in Rasch analyses is to construct simple scatterplots of residuals or standardized residuals associated with an item, person, or other element of interest. These plots illustrate the magnitude and direction of standardized residuals to supplement numeric fit statistics and provide additional insight into the nature of misfit for individual items or persons.

Item Separation on Latent Variable

In looking at the item locations on the variable map, it is important to have a range of values that serve to define the latent variable. It is important to address the following question:

- Are item locations spread out on the latent variable?

The spread of item locations on the latent variable provides evidence that the items reflect different levels of the construct and support meaningful person estimation at each level. The reliability of item separation statistic can be considered in conjunction with the substantive interpretation of item content based on the variable map. The reliability of item separation can be defined as follows:

$$\mathrm{REL_i} = (\mathrm{OV_i} - \mathrm{EV_i})/\mathrm{OV_i}$$

where $\mathrm{OV_i}$ = observed variance of item difficulty measures and $\mathrm{EV_i}$ = mean of squared standard errors of item difficulty measures.

Structural Aspects: Item Covariates

Structural aspects related to item covariates reflect a transition from evaluation criteria for descriptive Rasch models to an examination of model-data fit issues for explanatory Rasch models. Item covariates can be included to answer the following question:

How well do the item classifications predict item locations?

For example, the Linear Logistic Rasch Model (LLRM) can be used to model item locations based on item covariates. The item covariates can be categorical or continuous. The covariates reflect independent variables that can be used to explain variation in item locations. For example, item difficulty may be predicted by the level of a cognitive domain required to answer the item correctly. This extended Rasch model is introduced later in the book.

Person Focus

Since a major purpose of assessment includes the estimation and use of person scores, it is important to evaluate the psychometric quality of person responses. In this case, the questions mirror the ones posed for examining items:

- Are the person locations reasonable?
- Are persons associated with unexpected responses?
- Are person response functions monotonically decreasing on the latent variable?
- Are person locations spread out on the latent variable?

Person Locations

- Are the person locations reasonable?

As was the case with items, it is important to explore theoretical justifications for person locations on the variable map. For example, researchers should consider whether there are meaningful differences with respect to the latent variable between persons with different locations. Researchers should consider other sources of information to provide a theoretical justification for person locations on the latent variable. Qualitative data can also provide support for person locations on the latent variable. Demographic characteristics and other variables can provide evidentiary support for the meaning and use of the scores.

Person Fit

Person fit can be evaluated using the residuals described earlier, with residuals summarized for individual persons rather than items. Guiding questions for person fit analysis are:

- Are persons associated with unexpected responses?
- Are person response functions monotonically decreasing on the latent variable?

As was the case with item fit, several indices can be used to evaluate person fit:

- Infit/Outfit *MSE*
- Fit categories (A, B, C, D)
- Person response functions (graphical displays)

The person Infit and Outfit statistics can be calculated in a similar way to item fit statistics. Outfit *MSE* is calculated as the unweighted average of the standardized residuals associated with responses to the person of interest:

$$\textit{Outfit MSE} = \sum_{i=1}^{I} Z_{\mathrm{A}i}^2 / I, \tag{4.6}$$

where I is the number of observed responses for person A. As we saw for items, Infit *MSE* statistics are an alternative residual summary statistic similar to outfit *MSE* that are weighted by response variance to reduce the impact of outliers. Infit *MSE* for Person A is calculated as:

$$\textit{Infit MSE} = \sum_{i=1}^{I} W_{\mathrm{A}i} Z_{\mathrm{A}i}^2 / \sum_{I=1}^{I} W_{\mathrm{A}i}. \tag{4.7}$$

Person response functions can be evaluated by examining the observed and expected person response functions. Plots of these person response functions provide a useful graphical display for examining person fit. These plots typically include the expected person response function based on the measurement model with empirical data included to show model-data fit.

Person Separation on the Latent Variable

It is important to have a range or distribution of persons on the latent variable. The underlying question is:

- Are person locations spread out on the latent variable?

Similar to separation for items, person separation on the latent variable provides evidence that the measurement procedure was effective in identifying differences between individual persons with respect to the latent variable. It is possible to examine the reliability of person separation index in a manner similar to reliability of item separation. Reliability of person separation can be calculated as:

$$\mathrm{REL_p} = \left(\mathrm{OV_p} - \mathrm{EV_p}\right)/\mathrm{OV_p}$$

where $\mathrm{OV_p}$ = observed variance of person location measures and $\mathrm{EV_p}$ = mean of squared standard errors of person location measures. When there is adequate fit for items and persons, reliability of person separation statistics can be interpreted in a comparable way as coefficient alpha estimates of internal consistency from classical test theory.

Structural Aspects: Person Covariates

Structural aspects are not included in the dichotomous Rasch model described in this chapter. However, as was the case with items, the person scores can be examined within extended Rasch models, such as the Latent Regression Rasch Model. The key question is:

- How well do person categories predict person locations?

Extended Rasch models that include person covariates are introduced later in the book.

Illustration: Learning Stimulation Scale

In this section, we use data from the Learning Stimulation Scale introduced in Chap. 1 to illustrate the fit analysis procedures described in the previous sections. All analyses were conducted using the TAM and EIRM packages in R using marginal maximum likelihood estimation. Table 4.1 describes aspects of model-data fit related to Rasch measurement theory that are used as a guide in this section.

The first step is to load and prepare the data for analysis:

```
library(tam)
data <- read.csv("Homewide.csv", header = TRUE)
home.items <- data[,3:13]
```

Next, marginal maximum likelihood estimates of the item parameters are obtained using the tam.mml() function, which applies the dichotomous Rasch model.

```
Home <-tam.mml(home.items, verbose = FALSE)
summary(Home)
```

It should be noted that the item locations can be based on item easiness or difficulty.

Construct Focus

This section illustrates aspects of model-data fit that have a construct focus using the Learning Stimulation Scale.

Variable Map

After the Rasch model is estimated using TAM, a variable map can be displayed using the IRT.WrightMap() function:

```
IRT.WrightMap(Home,show.thr.lab=FALSE,     main.title     =
"Learning Stimulation Scale")
```

The variable map for the Learning Stimulation Scale is shown in Table 4.2 (Panel A).

Unidimensionality

Next, the unidimensionality of the Learning Stimulation Scale is examined. The indices in this section are based on residuals. Using TAM to fit the model as shown above, the expected responses and residuals can be extracted from the model results as follows:

```
Observed <- Home$resp
Residuals <- IRT.residuals(Home)
Expected <- Residuals$X_exp
resids.raw <- as.matrix(Observed-Expected)
```

Table 4.2 Construct focus for learning stimulation scale

1.1 Variable Maps

Panel A	Panel B
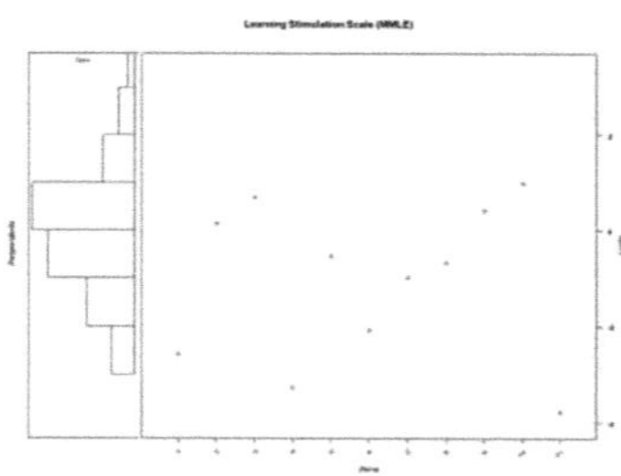	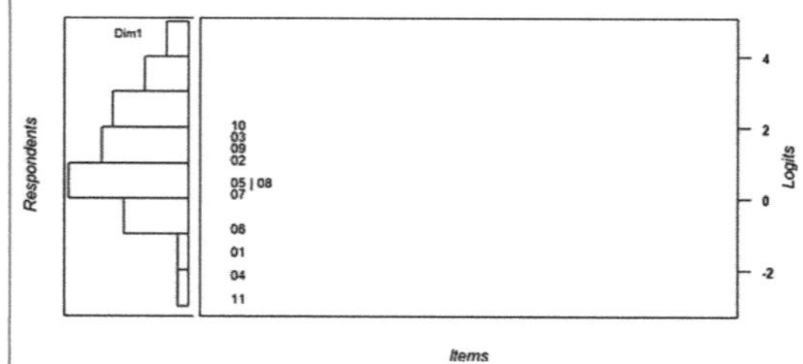

1.2 Unidimensionality

Percent of variance explained by model:
46.9%

Inter-item correlations of residuals: Table 4.3

Principal components analysis of residuals (First five eigenvalues):
2.15, 1.97, 1.60, 1.20, 0.98

Local independence (Mean with *SD* in parentheses):
Q3=−0.064 (0.175), aQ3=0.000(0.175)

1.3 Overall Model-data fit

Models	R Syntax	Npar	AIC	BIC	logLik	Deviance	Chisq	Df
Base	Rating ~ (1 | Person)	2	552	560	−274	548		
Rasch	Rating ~ −1 + item + (1 | Person)	12	451	500	−213	427	121*	10

* $p < 0.05$

```
Observed.vector <- as.vector(as.matrix(Observed))
Residuals.vector <- as.vector(resids.raw)
VO <- var(Observed.vector)
VR <- var(Residuals.vector)
# Variance explained by model
(VO-VR)/VO
```

The proportion of variance explained by the model is .469 (46.9%). Values greater than 20% are typically considered as evidence of acceptable unidimensionality for practical purposes (Reckase, 1979).

Next, the inter-item correlations for the residuals can be examined for evidence related to local independence. These residual correlations are shown in Table 4.3. A histogram of the residual correlations is shown in Fig. 4.2.

One popular method for evaluating local independence is the Q3 statistic proposed by Yen (1984). Q3 is based on the residual correlations, and we interpreted the values of Q3 according to guidance from Christensen, et al. (2017). Reflecting Christensen et al.'s general recommendations, inter-item residual correlations that exceed 0.20 above the average inter-item residual correlations may indicate local dependence. Again, it is important to consider all sources of evidence in conjunction with one another. These statistics for detecting local dependence can be calculated using functions from TAM:

```
##### Residual Correlations
Library (psych)
res1 <- TAM::tam.modelfit( tamobj=Home )
```

Table 4.3 Inter-item correlations of residuals: (aQ3)

	I1	I2	I3	I4	I5	I6	I7	I8	I9	I10	I11
I1	1.00	0.26	−0.23	0.29	0.13	0.32	−0.05	−0.09	−0.31	0.15	−0.37
I2	0.26	1.00	−0.27	0.12	−0.08	0.17	0.18	−0.12	0.11	−0.21	−0.22
I3	−0.23	−0.27	1.00	0.09	0.09	−0.26	−0.11	0.22	−0.11	0.12	0.08
I4	0.29	0.12	0.09	1.00	0.15	−0.16	−0.13	0.16	−0.11	0.06	0.19
I5	0.13	−0.08	0.09	0.15	1.00	−0.26	0.11	−0.15	−0.30	0.26	0.14
I6	0.32	0.17	−0.26	−0.16	−0.26	1.00	−0.01	0.13	0.03	−0.18	0.04
I7	−0.05	0.18	−0.11	−0.13	0.11	−0.01	1.00	−0.19	0.07	0.10	0.17
I8	−0.09	−0.12	0.22	0.16	−0.15	0.13	−0.19	1.00	−0.05	−0.09	0.14
I9	−0.31	0.11	−0.11	−0.11	−0.30	0.03	0.07	−0.05	1.00	−0.22	0.13
I10	0.15	−0.21	0.12	0.06	0.26	−0.18	0.11	−0.09	−0.22	1.00	0.06
I11	−0.37	−0.22	0.08	0.19	0.14	0.04	0.17	0.14	0.13	0.06	1.00
Mean	0.01	−0.01	−0.04	0.07	0.01	−0.02	0.01	0.00	−0.07	0.01	0.04
SD	0.25	0.20	0.18	0.15	0.19	0.20	0.13	0.15	0.16	0.17	0.18

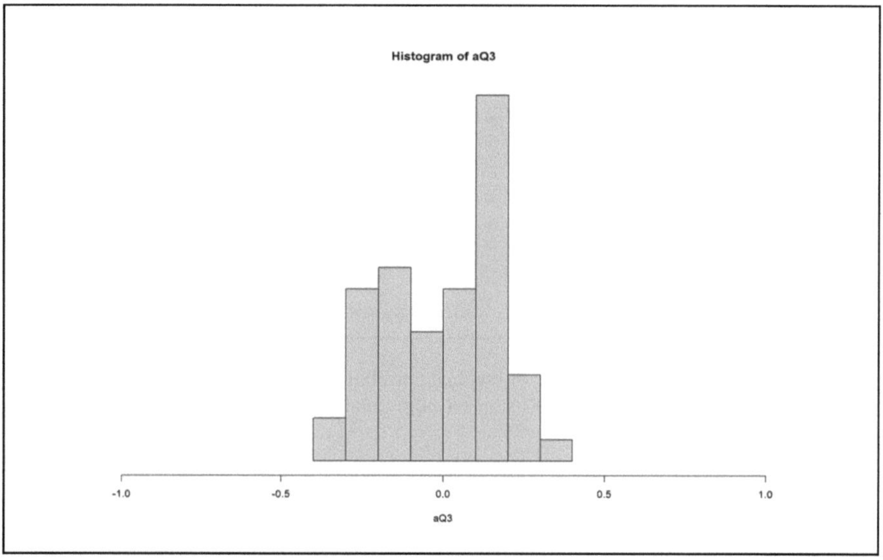

Fig. 4.2 Distribution of residual correlations

```
ResCorr <- res1[["Q3.matr"]]
adjResCorr <- res1[["aQ3.matr"]]
adjResCorr
#### Local Independence (aQ3)
aQ3 <- adjResCorr
describe(aQ3)
hist(aQ3,xlim=c(-1,1))
```

In these data, the minimum Q3 statistic is .223, the maximum aQ3 statistic is .319, the mean for the Q3 statistic is −0.064 (*SD* = 0.1752), and the mean for adjusted (aQ3) statistic is 0.000 (SD = 0.1752). There were two item pairs identified by the aQ3 values for the Learning Stimulation Scale as being statistically significant. Item 1 (Toys—Color and Shape) had the largest adjusted Q3 statistic with Item 11 (Shape Learning): aQ31,4 = −0.37. The second highest value was between Item 1 and Item 6 (Toys—teach numbers): aQ31,6 = .32. The strong association between these three items may reflect similar content in shape or number-related toys.

```
Nitems <- ncol(Observed)
pca <- pca(Residuals$stand_residuals,nfactors=Nitems,
rotate="none")
pca$values
contrasts <- c(pca$values[1:5])
plot(contrasts, ylab = "Eigenvalues for Contrasts", xlab =
"Contrast Number",
```

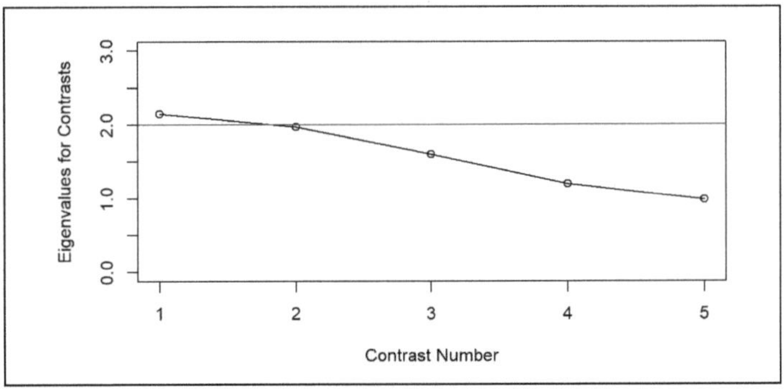

Fig. 4.3 Principal component analysis of residual correlations. *Note* Recommended critical value is 2.00—eigenvalues greater than 2.00 suggest additional potential dimensions in the residual correlations

```
main = "Contrasts from PCA of Standardized Residual Correla-
tions", col = "black")
lines(contrasts, col = "black")
abline(h = 2, col = "red")
```

To explore dimensionality, principal components analysis can also be conducted based on the residuals. We have found it useful to plot the first five eigenvalues. This is shown in Fig. 4.3 that presents the plots for the first five eigenvalues. The PCA-R indicates that there is one eigenvalue greater than 2.00, and this is the eigenvalue for the first contrast (2.15). An examination of the loadings on this first contrast suggests that Item 4 (free expression toys) had the largest loading on the first contrast (loading = 0.57).

Overall Model-Data Fit

Another source of evidence related to the overall construct is a comparison of model-data fit for the Rasch model with a base model using information statistics. In some cases, a likelihood ratio test for the difference between the two models can be conducted. To evaluate overall model-data fit, we use functions from the EIRM package in R. The EIRM package is used for explanatory Rasch models later in this chapter. In order to apply functions from the EIRM package, the data has to be changed from wide to long format. The following R code can be used for this purpose:

```
library(reshape2)
```

```
library(eirm)
data <- read.csv("Homewide.csv", header = TRUE)
head(data)
longdata  <-  melt(data,  id.vars=c("Person","Education"),
variable.name = "Item",
value.name = "Response")
head(longdata)
```

In this case, we are including "Education" as a person (in this case, home) covariate. The items in the Learning Stimulation Scale are classified as relating to child or adult objects as follows:

```
longdata$Class<- case_when(longdata$Item %in% c("I1", "I4",
"I5","I6","I7","I11") ~ "Child", longdata$Item %in% c("I2",
"I3", "I8","I9","I10") ~ "Adult")
longdata$Class <- as.character(longdata$Class)
longdata$Education <- as.character(longdata$Education)
head(longdata)
```

This defines the item covariate in the model.

Syntax representing the base model is "Response~(1|Person)"; this specification indicates that persons are a random effect. The R syntax for the base model is as follows:

```
Base <- eirm(formula = "Response~(1|Person)", data = long-
data)
summary(Base$model)
```

The R syntax for the Rasch model within EIRM is as follows:

```
Rasch <- eirm(formula = "Response~-1+Item+(1|Person)", data
= longdata)
print(Rasch, difficulty = TRUE) # To get difficulty parameters
summary(Rasch$model,corr=FALSE)
plot(Rasch,difficulty=TRUE) # Wright Map
```

The two models can be compared using the anova() function:

```
anova(Base$model, Rasch$model)
```

The analysis of overall model-data fit is shown in Table 4.2. The Rasch model has smaller values for all of the information indices. The base model in EIRM syntax is defined as: Rating ~ (1 | Person), while the Rasch model is defined as: Rating ~ −1 + Item + (1 | Person). The difference in the deviance statistics is distributed as a chi-squared statistic. The difference between the models is statistically significant with Chi-squared = 121 (df = 10).

Item Focus

Next, we examine the item locations using the variable map for the Learning Stimulation Scale as shown in Table 4.2 (Panel B). The ordering of the items seems to make sense—it is generally easier to observe child-related items as compared to adult-related items. It also makes sense that these homes have a relatively high level of learning stimulation. If possible, it would be useful to add qualitative information regarding this ordering of the home environments. There is evidence to support the inference that the Learning Stimulation Scale represents the intended construct.

Once the items are calibrated, several methods can be used to evaluate item fit. These include an examination of Infit and Outfit *MSE* statistics. The item-level fit statistics are shown in Table 4.4 (Panel A). The expected value for these statistics is 1.00. None of the absolute values of the standardized t-statistics are greater than 2.00, and this suggests that there is acceptable model-data fit for all of the items.

```
library(psych)
Items <- data.frame(Home$item_irt$beta,Home$se.AXsi)
summary(Items)
describe(Items[,c(1,3)])
```

The Outfit statistics can also be classified within fit categories using the dplyr package:

```
library(dplyr)
Items%>%
mutate(FitCategory=case_when(
Outfit >= .5 ~ "A",
Outfit > 1.5 ~ "B",
Outfit < .5 ~ "C",
Outfit > 2.0 ~ "D",
))
```

Nine of the items are in fit categories A (productive for measurement) or B (less productive but not distorting measures).

Table 4.4 Summary statistics for dichotomous rasch model: Learning stimulation scale

Panel A		Panel B	
2.0 Item focus		3.0 person focus	
2.1 Item locations		3.1 person locations	
Measures		Measures	
M	0.00	*M*	1.06
SD	1.64	*SD*	1.24
N	11	*N*	40
2.2 Item fit		3.2 person fit	
Outfit *MSE*		Outfit *MSE*	
M	0.89	*M*	0.71
SD	0.12	*SD*	0.54
Fit category	A=9, B=2, C=0, D=0	Fit category	A=17, B=17, C=4, D=2
Infit *MSE*		Infit *MSE*	
M	0.99	*M*	0.86
SD	0.12	*SD*	0.41
Fit category	A=11, B=0, C=0, D=0	Fit category	A=32, B=5, C=3, D=0
2.3 Reliability of item separation	0.904	3.3 Reliability of person separation	0.742
2.4 Item covariates	None	3.4 person covariates	None

Note The fit categories are defined as follows: (A) productive for measurement ($0.50 \leq MSE \leq 1.50$); (B) less productive but not distorting measures ($MSE < 0.50$); (C) unproductive but not distorting measures ($1.50 \leq MSE < 2.00$); and (D) unproductive and distorting measures ($MSE > 2.00$)

IRFs that include both model-expected and empirical responses are useful for visualizing model-data fit for each item. Figure 4.4 shows these plots for the 11 items included in the Learning Stimulation Scale. These plots can be generated as follows:

```
par(mfrow = c(3, 4))
plot(Home, items=1:11, export=FALSE)
Items <- data.frame(Home$item_irt$beta,Home$se.AXsi)
summary(Items)
describe(Items[,c(1,3)])
```

The reliability of item separation can be calculated as follows:

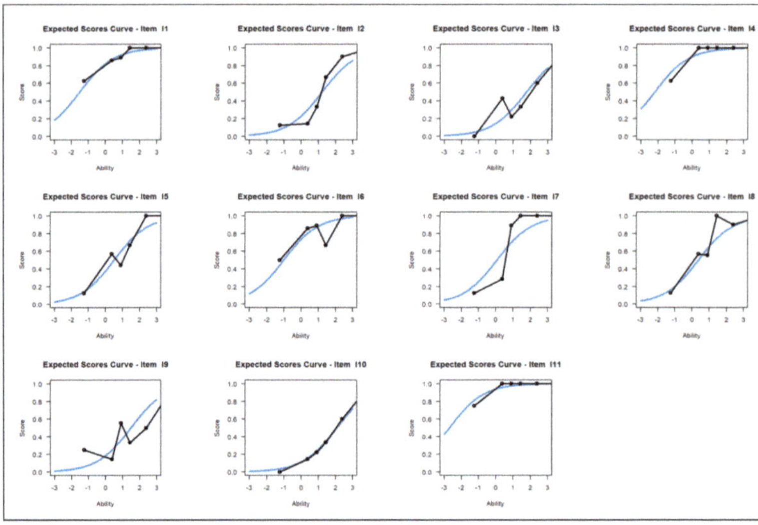

Fig. 4.4 Item fit plots for learning stimulation scale

```
OV <- var(Items[,1]) # Observed variance
EV <- sum(Items[,3]^2)/nrow(Items) # Expected variance
ItemReliability <- (OV-EV)/OV # Reliability of item separation
ItemReliability
```

The reliability of item separation is .904. This supports our conclusion about item spread on the latent variable based on the Wright map. It is important to note that child-related items are relatively easier to endorse as compared to adult-related items. There is evidence to support the inference of good psychometric quality of the items.

Person Focus

```
Persons <- data.frame(Home$person$EAP, Home$person$SD.EAP)
summary(Persons)
describe(Persons)
```

In Fig. 4.5, we plot several illustrative residual analyses related to persons (in this case, homes). The x-axis shows individual homes, and the y-axis shows the values of the standardized residuals. Dashed horizontal lines are plotted at $Z_{ni} = 2.00$ and $Z_{ni} = -2.00$ to indicate standardized residuals that are more than two standard deviations from the mean and indicate substantial departures from model expectations. The plots for Items 1 and 9 can be generated as follows:

```
#Item 1
plot(Residuals$stand_residuals[,1],ylim          =          c(-3,
3),xlab="Persons")
abline(h=c(-2,2),lty = 2)
#Item 9
```

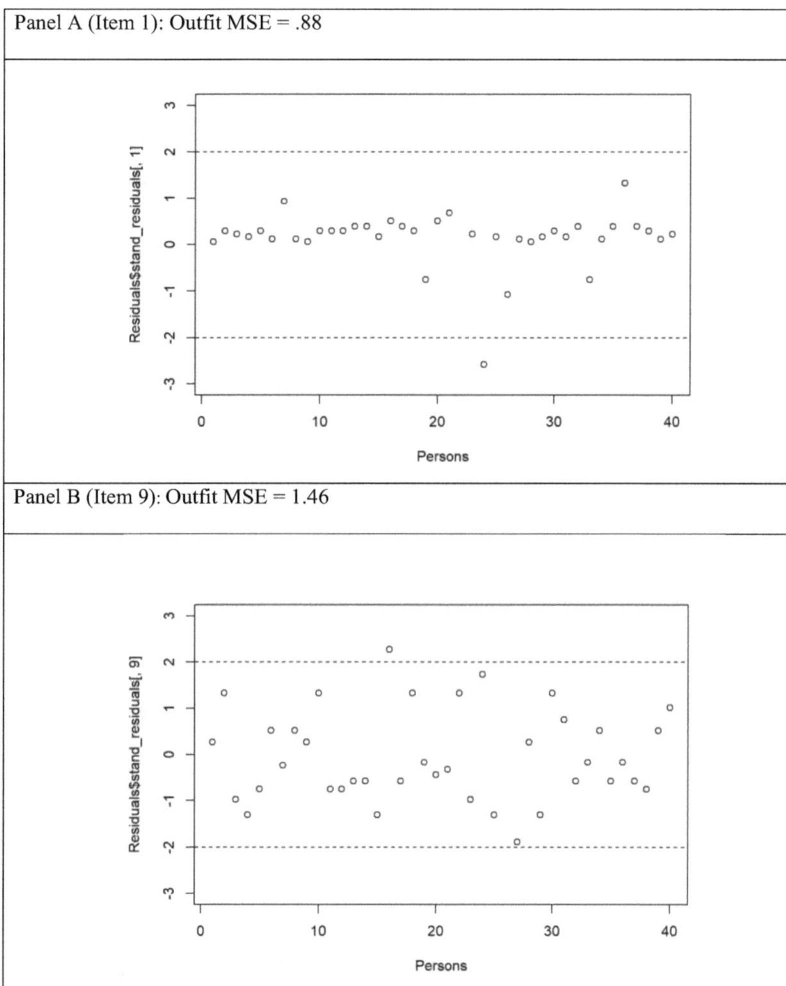

Fig. 4.5 Scatterplots of standardized residuals for selected items

```
plot(Residuals$stand_residuals[,9],ylim = c(-3,
3),xlab="Persons")
abline(h=c(-2,2),lty = 2)
```

On average, the person fit statistics indicated that responses for most homes reflected model expectations with average values of Infit *MSE* ($M = 0.86$) and Outfit *MSE* ($M = 0.71$) near 1.00. Table 4.5 presents summary statistics for each home environment. There only two homes in category D (unproductive for measurement, distorting of measures) based on Outfit *MSE*: Homes 24 and 26. Figure 4.6 shows a scatterplot of standardized residuals for Home 24. This can be plotted as follows:

```
# Standardized Person Residuals
# Person 24
plot(Residuals$stand_residuals[24,],ylim = c(-3, 3),xlab =
"Items")
abline(h=c(-2,2),lty = 2)
```

The reliability of person separation can be calculated as follows (Table 4.6):

```
Relperson <- Home$EAP.rel
```

Table 4.5 Summary statistics for items (Learning Stimulation Scale)

			Outfit			Infit		
Item	Location	*SE*	*MSE*	t-value	Fit category	*MSE*	t-value	Fit category
1	2.58	0.59	0.88	0.17	A	0.99	0.09	A
2	−0.14	0.42	1.00	0.08	A	0.95	−0.28	A
3	−0.71	0.43	1.10	0.38	A	1.11	0.68	A
4	3.26	0.72	0.34	−0.25	B	0.82	−0.26	A
5	0.55	0.43	0.87	−0.31	A	0.97	−0.11	A
6	2.08	0.53	1.11	0.39	A	1.10	0.45	A
7	1.00	0.44	0.73	−0.61	A	0.87	−0.68	A
8	0.70	0.43	1.04	0.22	A	0.98	−0.08	A
9	−0.42	0.42	1.46	1.40	A	1.26	1.52	A
10	−1.01	0.44	0.89	−0.14	A	0.96	−0.14	A
11	3.76	0.85	0.38	0.08	B	0.94	0.09	A

Note Locations are based on item easiness. A: 0.50<*MSE*<1.50 (Productive for measurement), B: *MSE*<0.50 (Less productive for measurement, but not distorting of measures), C: 1.50<*MSE*<2.00 (Unproductive for measurement, but not distorting of measures), D: *MSE*>2.00 (Unproductive for measurement, distorting of measures)

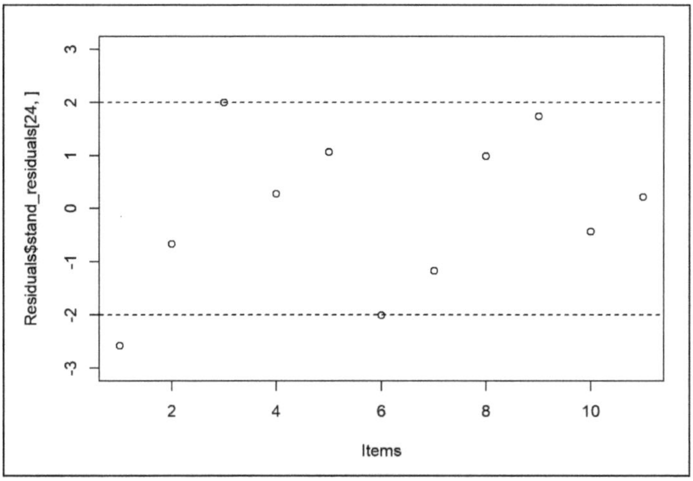

Fig. 4.6 Scatterplots of standardized residuals for home 24 (misfitting, Outfit MSE = 2.00)

The reliability of person separation statistic is .742. This value can be interpreted similarly to coefficient alpha in classical test theory. This value supports the visual evidence presented in the Wright maps (Figs. 1.3 and 4.1). There is evidence to support the conclusion that the homes can be located in a meaningful way on the construct.

Discussion and Summary

This chapter has focused on evaluating measurement quality for the dichotomous Rasch model. Good model-data fit is essential to achieve the desirable measurement qualities of Rasch measurement theory related to invariance.

Measurement quality can be evaluated using analyses of residuals. We described several indicators of measurement quality, organized around three aspects of model-data fit: Construct focus, item focus, and person focus. These indicators should be viewed in combination to support inferences about measurement quality based on the use of Rasch measurement theory within the context of particular scale administered to persons. It is important to remember that the model embodies the principles of invariant measurement, but model-data fit provides the evidentiary basis to support the hypothesis that invariant measurement has been achieved with a particular context. Rasch used the term “specific objectivity” to stress this idea, and it may be appropriate to also conceive of specific invariance in the same sense.

The Learning Stimulation Scale was introduced in Chap. 1, and we used it in this chapter to illustrate the calculation and interpretation of various model-data fit indices. We used two R programs (TAM and EIRM) to estimate the Rasch model,

Table 4.6 Summary statistics for homes (Learning Stimulation Scale)

Home	Home (EAP)	Home (SD.EAP)	Outfit *MSE*	Outfit t-value	Outfit Category	Infit *MSE*	Infit t-value	Infit Category
1	3.22	0.89	0.04	0.85	B	0.08	−0.78	B
2	0.97	0.67	0.55	−0.43	A	0.75	−0.76	A
3	1.43	0.69	0.38	−0.46	B	0.55	−1.56	A
4	1.93	0.73	0.59	0.13	A	0.99	0.10	A
5	0.97	0.67	1.52	0.83	C	1.56	1.59	C
6	2.51	0.79	0.36	0.28	B	0.74	−0.27	A
7	−0.86	0.70	1.80	1.03	C	1.41	0.96	A
8	2.51	0.79	1.13	0.75	A	1.11	0.38	A
9	3.22	0.89	0.04	0.85	B	0.08	−0.78	B
10	0.97	0.67	0.65	−0.26	A	0.86	−0.35	A
11	0.97	0.67	0.50	−0.54	A	0.67	−1.04	A
12	0.97	0.67	0.37	−0.83	B	0.48	−1.90	B
13	0.52	0.67	0.79	−0.16	A	0.93	−0.09	A
14	0.52	0.67	0.79	−0.16	A	0.93	−0.09	A
15	1.93	0.73	0.41	−0.07	B	0.70	−0.71	A
16	0.07	0.67	0.77	−0.26	A	0.78	−0.45	A
17	0.52	0.67	0.42	−1.01	B	0.55	−1.42	A
18	0.97	0.67	0.71	−0.16	A	0.98	0.03	A
19	−1.36	0.72	0.50	−0.06	A	0.91	−0.04	A
20	0.07	0.67	0.42	−1.16	B	0.54	−1.25	A
21	−0.38	0.68	0.62	−0.47	A	0.79	−0.38	A
22	0.97	0.67	1.75	1.04	C	1.44	1.30	A
23	1.43	0.69	1.66	0.88	C	1.40	1.20	A
24	0.52	0.67	2.00	1.46	D	1.98	2.29	C
25	1.93	0.73	0.47	0.00	B	0.81	−0.40	A
26	−0.86	0.70	2.31	1.40	D	1.78	1.56	C
27	2.51	0.79	0.45	0.36	B	0.84	−0.07	A
28	3.22	0.89	0.04	0.85	B	0.08	−0.78	B
29	1.93	0.73	0.41	−0.07	B	0.70	−0.71	A
30	0.97	0.67	0.71	−0.16	A	0.98	0.03	A
31	1.93	0.73	0.36	−0.14	B	0.61	−1.04	A
32	0.52	0.67	0.42	−1.01	B	0.55	−1.42	A
33	−1.36	0.72	0.25	−0.45	B	0.46	−1.30	B
34	2.51	0.79	0.36	0.28	B	0.74	−0.27	A
35	0.52	0.67	0.92	0.08	A	0.98	0.05	A
36	−1.36	0.72	0.73	0.19	A	1.38	0.88	A

(continued)

Table 4.6 (continued)

Home	Home (EAP)	Home (SD.EAP)	Outfit *MSE*	Outfit t-value	Outfit Category	Infit *MSE*	Infit t-value	Infit Category
37	0.52	0.67	0.64	−0.45	A	0.85	−0.33	A
38	0.97	0.67	0.73	−0.12	A	0.92	−0.15	A
39	2.51	0.79	0.29	0.20	B	0.61	−0.53	A
40	1.43	0.69	0.58	−0.14	A	0.82	−0.48	A

and to calculate indices described in this chapter. Future chapters extend these measurement quality indicators to include explanatory Rasch models, as well as for polytomous data.

In summary, this chapter introduced model-data fit indices for use with the dichotomous Rasch model. These indices, as well as other evidence, will be discussed for explanatory Rasch models in forthcoming chapters.

References

Akaike, H. (1973). Information theory and an extension of the maximum likelihood principle. In B. N. Petrov & F. Csaki (Eds.), *Second international symposium on information theory* (pp. 267–281). Budapest: Academiai Kiado.

Baker, F., & Kim, S.-H. (2004). *Item response theory: Parameter estimation techniques* (2nd ed.). CRC Press.

Bond, T. G., Yan, Z., & Heene, M. (2020). Applying the Rasch model. In *Fundamental measurement in the human sciences* (4th ed.). Routledge.

Chen, J., de la Torre, J., & Zhang, Z. (2013). Relative and absolute fit evaluation in cognitive diagnosis modeling. *Journal of Educational Measurement, 50*, 123–140.

Chou, Y.-T., & Wang, W.-C. (2010). Checking dimensionality in item response models with principal component analysis on standardized residuals. *Educational and Psychological Measurement, 70*(5), 717–731. https://doi.org/10.1177/0013164410379322

Christensen, K. B., Makransky, G., & Horton, M. (2017). Critical values for Yen's Q3: Identification of local dependence in the Rasch model using residual correlations. *Applied Psychological Measurement, 41*(3), 178–194. https://doi.org/10.1177/0146621616677520

Cohen, A. S., & Cho, S. J. (2016). Information criteria. *Handbook of item response theory: Models, statistical tools, and applications.*

Engelhard, G. (2022). Focus article: The pillars of measurement wisdom. *Journal of Applied Measurement, 23*(3/4).

Engelhard, G., & Wang, J. (2021). *Rasch models for solving measurement problems* (Vol. 187). https://us.sagepub.com/en-us/nam/rasch-models-for-solving-measurement-problems/book267292

Engelhard, G., & Wind, S. A. (2018). *Invariant measurement with raters and rating scales: Rasch models for rater-mediated assessments.* Taylor & Francis.

Karabatsos, G. (2000). A critique of Rasch residual fit statistics. *Journal of Applied Measurement, 1*(2), 152–176.

Linacre, J. M. (1998). Structure in Rasch residuals: Why principal components analysis (PCA)? *Rasch Measurement Transactions, 12*(2), 636.

Linacre, J. M. (2003). Data variance: Explained, modeled and empirical. *Rasch Measurement Transactions, 17*(3), 942–943.
Linacre, J. M. (2020). *A user's guide to WINSTEPS MINISTEP Rasch-model computer programs* (4.7.0). winsteps.com.
Linacre, J. M., & Wright, B. D. (1994). Chi square fit statistics. *Rasch Measurement Transactions, 8*(2), 360.
Marais, I. (2013). Local dependence. In K. B. Christensen, S. Kreiner, & M. Mesbah (Eds.), *Rasch models in health* (pp. 111–130). Wiley.
McCullagh, P. (2019). *Generalized linear models.* Routledge.
Raiche, G. (2005). Critical eigenvalue sizes in standardized residual principal components analysis. *Rasch Measurement Transactions, 19*, 1012.
Rasch, G. (1977). On specific objectivity: An attempt at formalizing the request for generality and validity of scientific statements. *Danish Yearbook of Psychology, 14*, 58–94.
Reckase, M. D. (1979). Unifactor latent trait models applied to multifactor tests: Results and implications. *Journal of Educational Statistics, 4*, 207–230.
Schwarz, G. (1978). Estimating the dimension of a model. *The Annals of Statistics*, 461–464.
Seol, H. (2016). Using the bootstrap method to evaluate the critical range of misfit for polytomous Rasch fit statistics. *Psychological Reports, 118*(3), 937–956.
Smith, R. M. (2004). Fit analysis in latent trait models. In E. V. Smith & R. M. Smith (Eds.), *Introduction to Rasch measurement* (pp. 73–92). JAM Press.
Smith, R. M., & Plackner, C. (2009). The family approach to assessing fit in Rasch measurement. *Journal of Applied Measurement, 10*(4), 424–437.
Stigler, S. M. (2016). *The seven pillars of statistical wisdom.* Harvard University Press.
Vrieze, S. I. (2012). Model selection and psychological theory: A discussion of the differences between the Akaike information criterion (AIC) and the Bayesian information criterion (BIC). *Psychological Methods, 17*, 228–243. https://doi.org/10.1037/a0027127
Wasserman, L. (2010). *All of statistics: A concise course in statistical inference.* Springer.
Wind, S. A., & Schumacker, R. E. (2021). Exploring the impact of missing data on residual-based dimensionality analysis for measurement models. *Educational and Psychological Measurement, 81*(2), 290–318. https://doi.org/10.1177/0013164420939634
Wolfe, E. W. (2013). A bootstrap approach to evaluating person and item fit to the Rasch model. *Journal of Applied Measurement, 14*(1), 1–9.
Wright, B. D., & Masters, G. N. (1982). *Rating scale analysis: Rasch measurement.* MESA Press.
Wu, M., & Adams, R. J. (2013). Properties of Rasch residual fit statistics. *Journal of Applied Measurement, 14*(4), 339–355.
Yen, W. M. (1984). Effects of local item dependence on the fit and equating performance of the three-parameter logistic model. *Applied Psychological Measurement, 8*(2), 125–145. https://doi.org/10.1177/014662168400800201

Chapter 5
Explanatory Rasch Models: Linear Logistic Rasch Models and Latent Regression Rasch Models

*Measurement and explanation are not mutually exclusive (*De Boeck and Wilson, 2016, *p. 567).*

The purpose of this chapter is to describe two explanatory Rasch Models: the Linear Logistic Rasch Model and the Latent Regression Rasch Model. First, the Linear Logistic Rasch Model (LLRM) is presented. The LLRM is an explanatory Rasch model that includes item covariates. An earlier version of this model was called the linear logistic test model (LLTM) by Fischer (1973), and it also has close connections to the many-facet Rasch model (MFRM) developed by Linacre (1989). In this chapter, we consider how parameters for the LLRM in this chapter can be estimated using generalized linear mixed models (GLMMs). The second explanatory Rasch model discussed in this chapter is the latent regression Rasch model (LRRM). The LRRM includes person covariates. We will show how the parameters of the LRRM can also be estimated with generalized linear mixed models.

Figure 5.1 presents a concept map of the descriptive and explanatory Rasch models that are discussed in this book. The descriptive models include the Dichotomous Model and the Polytomous Models (Rating Scale Model and Partial Credit Model). The LLRM and LRRM are constructed by adding explanatory covariates to descriptive dichotomous or polytomous models. This chapter is organized as follows. First, we present the LLRM, and illustrate its estimation and interpretation using the Learning Stimulation Scale (dichotomous responses) which we examined in Chap. 3. We demonstrate the LLRM for polytomous responses using the Attitude Toward Censorship (ATC) Scale originally developed by Rosander and Thurstone (1931). This is followed by a description of the LRRM. The LRRM is illustrated with the ATC Scale using two person covariates (gender and education). This chapter concludes with a discussion and summary.

G. Engelhard and S. A. Wind, *Invariant Measurement with Explanatory Rasch Models in the Human Sciences*, https://doi.org/10.1007/978-3-032-08816-1_5

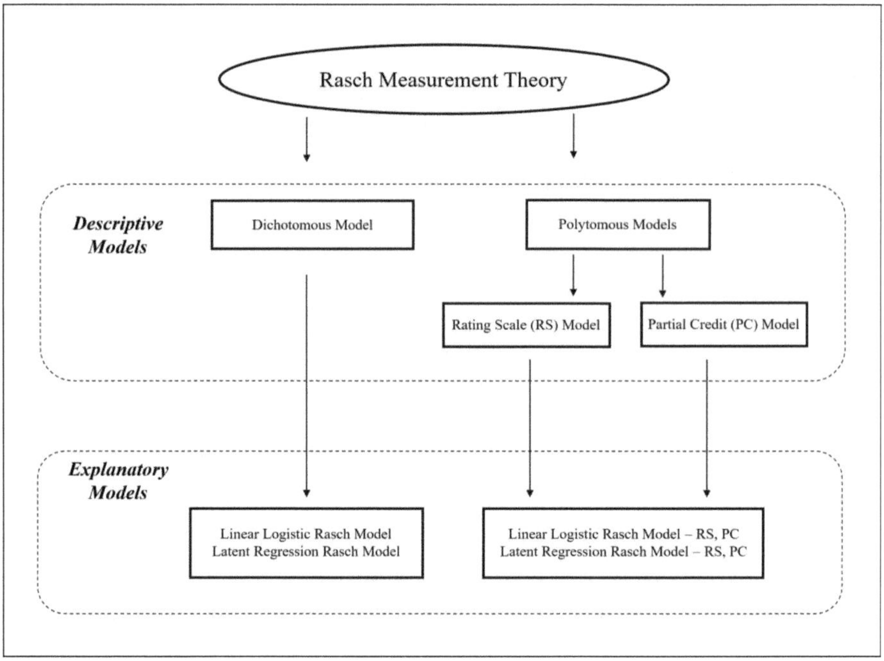

Fig. 5.1 Concept map for descriptive and explanatory models (dichotomous and polytomous data)

Table 5.1 First 10 cases for Learning Stimulation data files

Panel A: Wide format

	Person	I1	I2	I3	I4	I5	I6	I7	I8	I9	I10	I11
1	1	1	1	1	1	1	1	1	1	1	1	1
2	2	1	0	0	1	0	1	1	1	1	0	1
3	3	1	1	0	1	1	1	1	1	0	0	1
4	4	1	0	1	1	1	1	1	1	0	1	1
5	5	1	0	1	1	1	0	1	0	0	1	1
6	6	1	1	0	1	1	1	1	1	1	1	1
7	7	1	1	0	1	0	0	0	0	0	0	0
8	8	1	1	1	1	1	1	1	0	1	1	1
9	9	1	1	1	1	1	1	1	1	1	1	1
10	10	1	0	0	1	1	1	0	1	1	0	1

Panel B: Long format with item content

	Person	Item	Response	Content
1	1	I1	1	Child
2	2	I1	1	Child
3	3	I1	1	Child
4	4	I1	1	Child
5	5	I1	1	Child
6	6	I1	1	Child
7	7	I1	1	Child
8	8	I1	1	Child
9	9	I1	1	Child
10	10	I1	1	Child

Linear Logistic Rasch Model

Dichotomous Responses

De Boeck & Wilson (2004) distinguished between models within the family of Rasch models as descriptive or explanatory models. Descriptive models are defined by modeling both persons and items as fixed effects, with no additional explanatory variables. The Dichotomous Model, Rating Scale Model, and Partial Credit Model are prime examples of descriptive models. Explanatory models are defined by adding either item or person covariates to the model. The purpose of adding these covariates is to explain their influence on the probability of a response. These covariates can be modeled as random or fixed effects depending on the context of the assessment. The LLRM is an explanatory Rasch model with item covariates.

Parameters for explanatory Rasch models can be estimated with GLMMs. GLMMs can be viewed as consisting of three components: random component, linking component, and linear component. For example, the random component of the Dichotomous Model (DM) is

$$Y_{ni} \sim binomial(1, \pi_{ni}). \tag{5.1}$$

This represents the assumption that the observed responses, Y, are drawn from a binomial distribution with a probability of π_{ni}. The combination of binomial item responses yields a Bernoulli distribution.

The second component is called the linking component. The linking component serves to connect the probability of a response to a linear scale. For the Dichotomous Model, logits are typically used:

$$\eta_{ni} = \ln\left(\frac{\pi_{ni}}{1 - \pi_{ni}}\right). \tag{5.2}$$

This linking component connects the π_{ni} through a logistic transformation called logits (η_{ni}). For explanatory models, this linking component can be modeled with a linear component that includes covariates. Examples of other potential linking functions include the probit link function for binary data, and log link function for Poisson data.

The third component is the linear component that relates structural aspects of the model to the logits. The structural component may include covariates for persons and items as follows

$$\eta_{ni} = \boldsymbol{\theta}\mathbf{Z} - \boldsymbol{\beta}\boldsymbol{X} \tag{5.3}$$

where η_{ni} are logits, **Z** is a design matrix for persons, and **X** is a design matrix for items.

Following de Boeck et al. (2011), the linear component for the DM can be written as

$$\eta_{ni} = \theta Z_{i0} + \sum_{k=1}^{K} \beta_{1i} X_{ik} \tag{5.4}$$

with Z_{i0}= 1 for all items; X_{ik}= 1 if $i = k$ ($k = 1,\ldots,K$) and 0 otherwise, K is number of items, and.

θ ~ $N(0, \sigma_\theta^2)$. It should be noted that β is interpreted as item easiness in Eq. 5.4. The design matrix for persons (θ) consists of a indicator vector of 1s (Z = 1), and indicators for items. This is shown below for two persons and three items.

Person	Z	Item 1	Item 2	Item 3
1	1	1	0	0
1	1	0	1	0
1	1	0	0	1
2	1	1	0	0
2	1	0	1	0
2	1	0	0	1

As pointed out earlier, the basic formulation of LLRMs with GLMMs can be viewed as a random intercept model with persons (θ) as a random effect, and items (β) as fixed effects.

Conceptually, the LLRM can be viewed as including a structural model for explaining and predicting item difficulties using various covariates.

Illustration with Learning Stimulation Scale

In this section, we return to the Learning Stimulation Scale that has been discussed in other chapters. The responses are dichotomous for this scale. We use the EIRM package in R (Bulut, 2021) for the analyses in this section.

As is the case with all measurement models, including extended Rasch models, it is a good practice to begin measurement by focusing on the construct or latent variable. Explanatory Rasch models depend in a fundamental way on the theoretical conceptualization and empirical representation of the constructs, including their proposed relationships to other variables such as item covariates. A useful foundational question to begin a descriptive or extended Rasch model analysis is:

- What is the key construct in the model?

The LLRM focuses on item covariates. This focus on items requires researchers to identify item covariates to include in the model. When considering potential item-related covariates, researchers can ask: What are the domains or components that guided the creation of the items to represent the construct? For example, domains or components could represent learning objectives associated with items, levels within a taxonomy, visual features included in an item, or content classifications.

Results related to these domains can provide validity evidence regarding the interpretation and use of the scores. The following questions guide the identification and interpretation of covariates in an extended Rasch model context:

- What are the item covariates?
- How well do the item covariates predict item locations?

The item covariate for the Learning Stimulation Scale reflects the focus of the activities addressed in the items (child or adult activities).

To estimate the LLRM using the EIRM package, the first step is to read in the data, and convert it to long format:

```
rm(list=ls(all=TRUE))
library(eirm)
library(dplyr)
library(reshape2)
data <- read.csv("1 Learning Stimulation Scale Item Covari-
ates.csv", header = TRUE)
longdata <- melt(data, id.vars=c("Person"), variable.name =
"Item",
value.name = "Response")
```

Next, the item covariate (Content) is added to the wide data.

```
longdata$Content = case_when(longdata$Item %in% c("I1",
"I4", "I5","I6","I7","I11") ~ "Child", longdata$Item %in%
c("I2", "I3", "I8","I9","I10") ~ "Adult")
longdata$Content <- as.character(longdata$Content)
head(data)
head(longdata,10)
```

The re-shaped data are shown in Table 5.1. Panel A shows the data using wide format, and Panel B shows the data using long format, with the addition of the item content covariate.

Next, we estimate the LLRM as an item-covariates model. The EIRM syntax for the LLRM with item classification as a covariate is:

```
LLRM <- eirm(formula = "Response~-1+Content+(1|Person)",
data = longdata)
```

The following two commands can be used to obtain the mean item locations for each classification, and to plot the predicted probabilities:

Table 5.2 Estimates of item covariates (Learning Stimulation Scale)

	Item classification (LLRM)	
	η	*SE*
Item focus		
Content		
1. Adult (A)	−0.28	0.25
2. Child (C)	1.82	0.27

Note η is an average logit on the GLMM scale. LLRM is the Linear Logistic Rasch Model,

```
summary (LLRM$model)
marginalplot (LLRM, predictors = c("Content"))
```

As shown in Table 5.2, the mean item location for the adult items ($\eta = -0.28$, *SE* = 0.25) is lower than the mean location for the child items ($\eta = 1.82$, *SE* = 0.27). Higher values of η indicate higher probabilities of the activity being observed in the home, while lower values of η are associated with lower probabilities of occurrence in the home. The predicted probabilities are shown graphically in Fig. 5.2. The predicted probabilities provide a helpful tool for interpreting the results of the analyses. The results suggest that the activities reflected in the child items are easier to appear in a home environment as compared to the adult items. Adult items may reflect activities that are more costly to provide in the home or may reflect other characteristics, such as the educational level of the mother.

Polytomous Responses

Polytomous responses are widely used as the response format for many attitude scales. Popular polytomous descriptive Rasch models include the Rating Scale and Partial Credit Models (Engelhard & Wind, 2018). The evaluation of rating scale models is covered in detail in Chap. 8.

Following Stanke and Bulut (2019), the Partial Credit Model for adjacent response categories can be written as:

$$\ln\left[\frac{P(X_{nij} = 1)}{1 - P(X_{ni(j-1)} = 1)}\right] = \theta_n - (\delta_i + \tau_{ji}) \tag{5.5}$$

where X_{ni} is the observed response from person *n* on item *i*, θ_n is location of person *n* on the latent variable, δ_i is the location of item *i* on the latent variable, and τ_{ji} are the threshold parameters for adjacent categories. Eq. 5.5 can be modified to represent

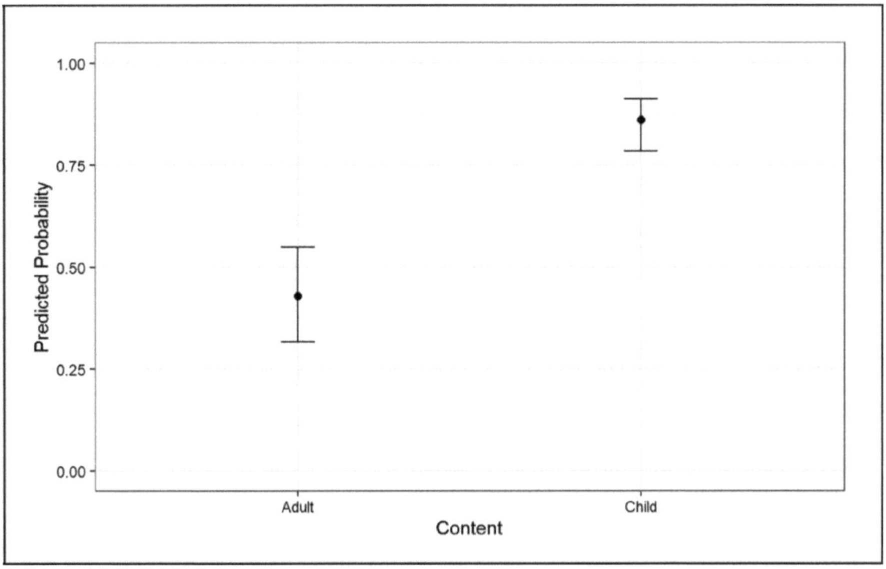

Fig. 5.2 Learning Stimulation Scale: Predicted probabilities for Item-Explanatory Rasch Model (Content Focus: Adult and Child Activities)

the Rating Scale Model (Andrich, 2016) by fixing the τ_{ji} to have the same values across items (τ_j).

The explanatory form of the Partial Credit Model (Stanke & Bulut, 2019; Tuerlinckx & Wang, 2004) can be written as

$$\ln\left[\frac{P(X_{nij}=1)}{1-P(X_{ni(j-1)}=1)}\right] = \mathbf{Z_n\theta_n} - \mathbf{X_i'\delta_i} + \tau_{ji} \tag{5.6}$$

where $\mathbf{Z_n}$ is a matrix of person covariates reflecting person characteristics, $\mathbf{X_i}$ is a matrix of item covariates that describes item characteristics.

Illustration with Attitude Toward Censorship Scale.

This illustration evaluates the ATC Scale using the LLRM. It differs from the previous illustration using the Learning Stimulation Scale because the responses are polytomous for the ATC Scale. The item covariate is item valence.

The key underlying construct on the ATC Scale is attitude toward censorship. According to the ACLU: "Censorship, the suppression of words, images, or ideas that are "offensive", happens whenever some people succeed in imposing their personal political or moral values on others. Censorship can be carried out by the government as well as private pressure groups" (https://www.aclu.org/documents/what-censorship). The items included in the ATC Scale are shown in Table 5.3. The ATC Scale was administered to a sample of adults ($N = 950$). Respondents were asked to rate their personal views of the 20 items using four categories: Strongly Disagree,

```
+---------------------------------------------+
|Logit|+Person     |-Items              |POLYS|
|-----+------------+--------------------+-----|
|     | *****.     |                    | (4) |
|     |            |                    |     |
|     | *.         |                    |     |
|     |            |                    |     |
|     | .          |                    |     |
|   2 +            +                    +     |
|     | *.         |                    |     |
|     | **.        |                    |     |
|     | ****.      |                    |     |
|     |            |                    | --- |
|     | **         |                    |     |
|     | **         |                    |     |
|     | *.         |                    |     |
|     | *.         |                    |     |
|     | **.        |                    |     |
|   1 + **.        +                    +     |
|     | **.        |                    |     |
|     | **.        |                    |     |
|     | **.        |                    |     |
|     | ******.    |                    |  3  |
|     | ***.       |                    |     |
|     | **.        | 9                  |     |
|     | ******.    | 10  7              |     |
|     | ***.       | 13  15  18  3   5  |     |
|     | ********   | 1   11  4          |     |
*   0 * ****.      * 19  6              *     *
|     | ********** | 14                 | --- |
|     | **.        | 12  16             |     |
|     | ******.    | 8                  |     |
|     | .          |                    |     |
|     | **         | 17  2   20         |     |
|     | .          |                    |     |
|     | .          |                    |  2  |
|     | .          |                    |     |
|     |            |                    |     |
|  -1 + .          +                    +     |
|     |            |                    |     |
|     | .          |                    |     |
|     | .          |                    |     |
|     |            |                    |     |
|     |            |                    | --- |
|     | .          |                    |     |
|     |            |                    |     |
|     |            |                    |     |
|  -2 +            +                    +     |
|     |            |                    |     |
|     |            |                    |     |
|     |            |                    |     |
|     |            |                    |     |
|     | .          |                    | (1) |
|-----+------------+--------------------+-----|
|Logit| * = 10     |-Items              |POLYS|
+---------------------------------------------+
```

Fig. 5.3 Variable Map for ATC Scale. *Note* Variable Map was created using the Facets Program (Linacre, 1989)

Disagree, Agree, or Strongly Agree. These ratings reflect the views of censorship by each participant on each item. The descriptive statistics for the sample are given in Table 5.4. The specific item covariate that is included in the explanatory model is valence.

Sentiment analysis was used to categorize the valence of the items in the ATC Scale. Sentiment analysis provides an approach for examining the emotional meaning of words in the attitude statements for respondents. Sentiment analysis was used to determine the valence of the attitude statements. The processes include the

Table 5.3 Attitude Toward Censorship scale

Item	Text	Mean	*SD*	Valence
1	I doubt if censorship is wise	2.85	.87	Neutral
2	A truly free people must be allowed to choose their own reading and entertainment	3.20	.81	Positive
3	We must have censorship to protect the morals of young people	2.79	.96	Positive
4	The theory of censorship is sound, but censors make a mess of it	2.84	.92	Negative
5	Only narrow-minded puritans want censorship	2.80	.96	Neutral
6	The whole theory of censorship is utterly unreasonable	2.88	.93	Neutral
7	Until public taste has been educated, we must continue to have censorship	2.75	.98	Positive
8	Many of our greatest literary classics would be suppressed if the censors thought they could get away with it	3.08	.81	Positive
9	Everything that is printed for publication should first be examined by government censors	2.68	1.05	Negative
10	Plays and movies should be censored but the press should be free	2.70	1.04	Neutral
11	Censorship has practically no effect on peoples morals	2.88	.91	Positive
12	Censorship is a gross violation of our constitutional right	3.02	.85	Negative
13	Censorship protects those who lack judgment or experience to choose for themselves	2.82	.94	Negative
14	Censorship is a very difficult problem, and I am not sure how far I think it should go	2.95	.90	Negative
15	Censorship is a good thing on the whole although it is often abused	2.82	.93	Positive
16	Education of the public taste is preferable to censorship	3.03	.85	Positive
17	Human progress demands free speech and a free press	3.19	.77	Positive
18	Censorship is effective in raising moral and aesthetic standards	2.78	.97	Positive
19	Censorship might be warranted if we could get reasonable censors	2.89	.92	Neutral
20	Morality is produced by self-control not by censorship	3.18	.80	Positive

Note This scale is from Rosander & Thurstone (1931). The observed ratings are defined as follows: 1 = Strongly Disagree, 2 = Disagree, 3 = Agree, and 4 = Strongly Agree. Valence was assigned based on sentiment analysis (Jockers, 2015)

Table 5.4 ATC scale: Description of the participants

	Frequency	Percentage
Gender		
1-male	499	52.5
2-female	451	47.5
College		
1-not a college graduate	229	24.1
2-college graduate	721	75.9
Age		
1–18–24	203	21.4
2–25–44	588	61.9
3–45–59	124	13.0
4–60 and older	35	3.7
Race/ethnicity		
1-white	792	83.4
2-black	27	2.8
3-Asian	50	5.3
4-other	81	8.5

Table 5.5 First 10 cases for ATC scale files

Panel A: Wide format

	Person	Gender	College	I1	I2	I3	I4	I5	I6	I7	I8	I9	I10	I11	I12	I13	I14	I15	I16	I17	I18	I19	I20
1	1	2	1	4	4	3	4	1	4	2	4	1	1	1	4	3	4	2	4	4	2	3	4
2	2	1	2	3	4	1	2	4	3	1	4	1	1	3	3	1	2	2	2	4	1	2	4
3	3	1	2	2	1	2	2	3	2	3	3	3	3	1	2	3	4	2	1	2	3	2	2
4	4	1	1	3	3	2	3	2	2	2	3	2	3	3	2	3	3	3	3	3	2	4	4
5	5	1	2	3	2	2	2	2	2	2	2	2	2	2	2	2	3	2	2	2	2	3	2
6	6	1	2	4	4	1	1	3	4	1	4	1	1	1	4	1	3	1	4	4	2	1	4
7	7	2	3	4	4	1	1	4	2	1	3	1	1	4	4	2	1	1	2	4	1	1	3
8	8	1	2	4	4	1	1	4	4	1	4	1	1	2	4	1	1	1	4	4	1	1	4
9	9	1	1	3	4	2	1	2	4	1	3	1	2	3	4	2	1	1	3	4	1	1	4
10	10	1	1	3	4	1	1	3	3	1	3	1	1	1	3	1	1	1	4	4	1	2	4

Panel B: Wide format with item valence

	Person	Gender	College	Item	Rating	Valence
1	1	2	1	I1	4	0
2	2	1	2	I1	3	0
3	3	1	2	I1	2	0
4	4	1	1	I1	3	0
5	5	1	2	I1	3	0
6	6	1	2	I1	4	0
7	7	2	3	I1	4	0
8	8	1	2	I1	4	0
9	9	1	1	I1	3	0
10	10	1	1	I1	3	0

categorization of the statements as having positive, negative, or neutral valences (Mohammad, 2016). The sentiment analyses in this study were conducted using the Syuzhet package in R (Jockers, 2015), and it is based on the NRC Emotion Lexicon. For example, the word "censor" creates a negative sentiment, while the word "free" creates a positive sentiment. Item 2 has a positive valence of 1: "truly free people must be allowed to choose their own reading and entertainment". On the other hand, Item 9 has a negative valence of −1: "Everything that is printed for publication should first be examined by government censors". The issue of valence becomes particularly important within the context of the measurement of attitudes toward controversial topics, such as abortion, the death penalty, and censorship.

The censorship data is read into R, and then converted using the polyreformat function (discussed further in chapter 8). Next, the item covariate (valence) is added to the file:

```
library(eirm)
library(dplyr)
library(lme4)
data <- read.table("Censorship (20 Items).csv", head=T,
sep=",")
censorlong <- melt(data = data,
# Student-level variables
id.vars = c("Person","Gender","College"),
# Item-level variables
measure.vars = paste0("I", c(1:20)),
# Name for the item labels in the long-format data
variable.name = "Item",
# Name for the responses in the long-format data
value.name = "Rating",
# Remove missing values in the items during reshaping
na.rm = TRUE)
censorlong2 <- polyreformat(data = censorlong,
id.var = c("Person", "Gender", "College"),
var.name = "Item",
val.name = "Rating")
censorlong2$Valence = case_when(censorlong$Item %in%
c("I1","I5", "I6", "I10","I19") ~ 0,
censorlong$Item %in% c("I2","I3","I7","I8","I11","I15") ~ 1,
censorlong$Item %in% c("I16","I17") ~ 1,
censorlong$Item %in% c("I18","I20") ~ 1,
censorlong$Item %in% c("I4") ~ -1,
censorlong$Item %in% c("I9","I12","I13","I14") ~ -1)
```

The re-shaped data are shown in Table 5.5. Panel A shows the data in wide format, and Panel B shows long format with item valences as a covariate. Education level and gender are also included in the data set, and they will be analyzed later in this chapter with the LRRM as person covariates.

Next, the model-data fit of the Rating Scale and Partial Credit Model can be compared. The Rating Scale and Partial Credit models are commonly used to model polytomous data, and it is important to consider which model provides the best fit to observed data, as well as substantive information for deciding on the appropriate model. The summary of the fit statistics is shown in Table 5.6. The following R syntax can be used to fit the two models:

```
#####
rsm <- eirm(formula = "polyresponse ~ -1 + Item + polycategory
+ (1|Person)",data = censorlong2)
summary(rsm$model)
marginalplot(rsm, predictors = c("Item"))
#####
pcm  <-  eirm(formula  =  "polyresponse  ~  -1  +  Item  +
Item:polycategory + (1|Person)",data = censorlong2)
summary(pcm$model)
marginalplot(pcm, predictors = c("Item"))
```

As shown in Table 5.6, the BIC statistic indicates that Rating Scale Model provides better model-data fit. The category response function for the RSM is shown in Fig. 5.4.

Using the Rating Scale Model, the EIRM syntax for the LLRM with item valence as a covariate is:

Table 5.6 ATC scale: Model-data fit summary (Linear Logistic Rasch Models)

	Fit statistics					
Models	BIC	AIC	Deviance	logLik	*df*	R Syntax
Rating scale models						
1. Rating scale model	39001.6	38810.0	38764.0	−19382.0	30,659	Polyresponse ~ −1 + item + polycategory + (1 I person)
2. Partial credit model	39240.5	38732.3	38610.3	−19305.2	30,621	Polyresponse ~ −1 + item + item:Polycategory + (1 I person)
Linear logistic Rasch model						
3. Valence	39090.3	39048.6	39038.6	−19519.3	30,677	Polyresponse ~ −1 + valence + polycategory + (1 I person)

Note BIC is used in this study for comparing models with smaller values of BIC indicating better model-data fit

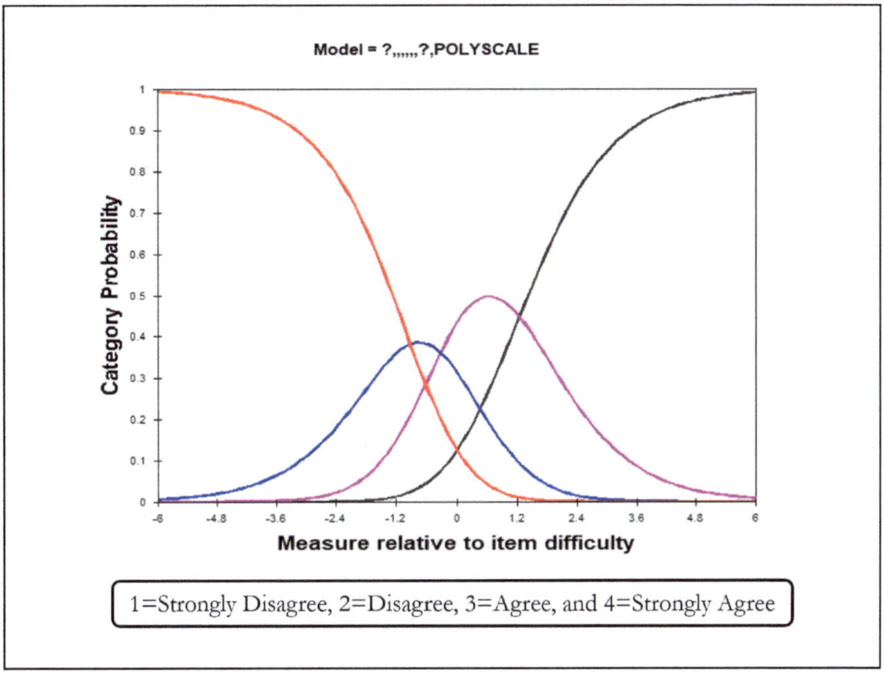

Fig. 5.4 ATC Scale: Category Response Function (Rating Scale Model). *Note* The category probability functions were created using the Facets Program (Linacre, 1989)

```
lltm_rsm <- eirm(formula = "polyresponse ~ -1 +
factor(Valence) + polycategory + (1|Person)", data =
censorlong2)
```

The following two commands can be used to obtain the mean item locations for each classification, and to plot the predicted probabilities:

```
summary(lltm_rsm$model)
marginalplot(lltm_rsm, predictors = c("Valence"))
```

The mean item location by valence is shown in Table 5.7. Higher values of η indicate higher probabilities associated with positive valences. The predicted probabilities by valence are shown graphically in Fig. 5.5. The data suggest that item valence is not a statistically significant predictor, although items with a positive valence tend to be easier to endorse.

Table 5.7 Estimates of item covariates (ATC Scale)

	Item classification (LLRM)	
	η	*SE*
Item focus		
Valence		
1 (positive)	1.42	.04
0 (neutral)	1.21	.04
–1 (negative)	1.26	.04

Note η is an average logit on the GLMM scale. LLRM is the Linear Logistic Rasch Model

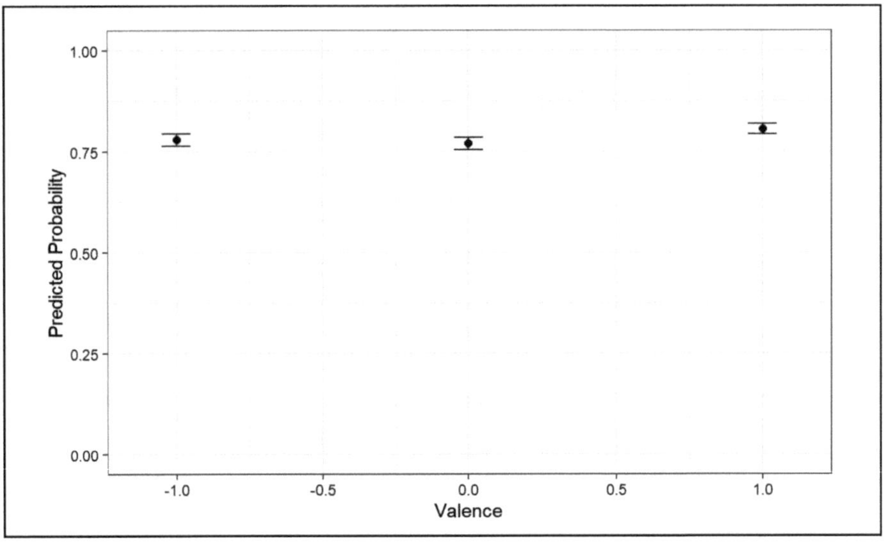

Fig. 5.5 ATC Scale: Predicted probabilities for Item-Explanatory Rasch Model (Focus: Valence). *Note* -1 = Negative valence, 0 = Neutral valence, 1 = Positive valence

Latent Regression Rasch Model

This section continues the analyses of the ATC Scale using the LRRM. The two person covariates are education level (not a college graduate/college graduate) and gender. These covariates are represented in the data as "College" and "Gender" respectively.

Illustration: Attitude Toward Censorship Scale (Continued).

The data have already been read into R with the data set called "censor_long2" used in this section. Using the Rating Scale Model, the EIRM syntax for the LRRM with College used as a person covariate is:

```
LRRM_rsm1 <- eirm(formula = "polyresponse ~ -1 + factor(College) +
polycategory + (1|Person)", data = censor_long2)
```

The following two commands can be used to obtain the mean person locations for each level of College, and to plot the predicted probabilities:

```
summary (LRRM_rsm1$model)
marginalplot(LRRM_rsm1,predictors = c("College"))
```

The mean person location by level of College is shown in Table 5.8. Higher values of η indicate higher probabilities associated with College graduates. The predicted probabilities by level of College are shown graphically in Fig. 5.6 (Panel A). The results suggest that College is a statistically significant predictor with College graduates indicating a higher level of support for censorship.

Next, Gender was included as a person covariate and mean locations for Gender including a plot of the predicted probabilities using the following EIRM syntax:

Table 5.8 ATC scale: Model-data fit summary (Latent Regression Rasch Models)

	Fit statistics					
Rating scale models	BIC	AIC	Deviance	logLik	*df*	R Syntax
1. Rating scale model	39001.6	38810.0	38764.0	−19382.0	30,659	Polyresponse ~ −1 + item + polycategory + (1 I person)
2. Partial credit model	39240.5	38732.3	38610.3	−19305.2	30,621	Polyresponse ~ −1 + item + item:Polycategory + (1 I person)
Latent regression Rasch model						
3. College	38980.2	38938.5	38928.5	−19464.3	30,677	Polyresponse ~ −1 + factor(college) + polycategory + (1 I person)
4. Gender	39096.8	39055.2	39045.2	−19522.6	30,677	Polyresponse ~ −1 + factor(gender) + polycategory + (1 I person)
5. College*gender	38987.8	38929.5	38915.5	−19,457	30,675	Polyresponse ~ −1 + college*gender + polycategory + (1 I person) Data: Data

Note BIC is used in this study for comparing models with smaller values of BIC indicating better model-data fit

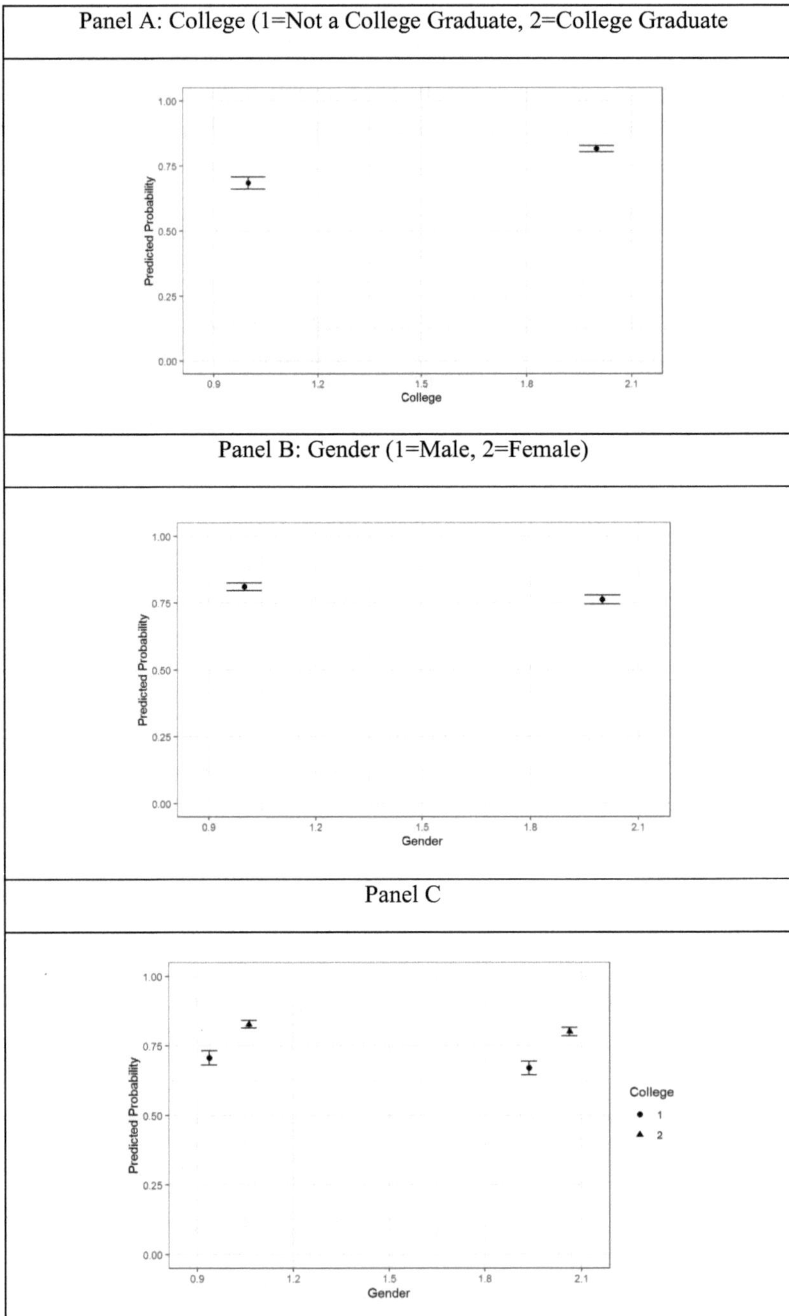

Fig. 5.6 ATC Scale: Predicted probabilities for Person-Explanatory Rasch Models (College and Gender)

Table 5.9 Estimates of person covariates (ATC Scale)

	η	*SE*
College		
No	0.77	0.06
Yes	1.49	0.04
Gender		
Male	1.45	0.05
Female	1.16	0.05

Note η is an average logit on the GLMM scale

```
LRRM_rsm2 <- eirm(formula = "polyresponse ~ -1 +
factor(Gender) + polycategory + (1|Person)", data = censor_
long2)
summary(LRRM_rsm2$model)
marginalplot(LRRM_rsm2, predictors = c("Gender"))
```

The mean person location by gender is shown in Table 5.9. Higher values of η indicate higher probabilities associated with male respondents. The predicted probabilities by gender are shown graphically in Fig. 5.6 (Panel B). The data suggest that gender is a statistically significant predictor with male respondents indicating a higher level of support for censorship.

The interaction between the two covariates (College and Gender) was examined using the following R code:

```
LRRM_rsm4 <- eirm(formula = "polyresponse ~ -1 +
Gender*College + polycategory + (1|Person)", data = censor_
long2)
summary(LRRM_rsm4$model) # Easiness order(Difficulty is what
we use)
marginalplot(LRRM_rsm4, predictors = c("Gender","College"
))
```

The analyses suggest that there is not a statistically significant interaction effect between College and Gender. College graduates support higher levels of censorship within Gender subgroups. The predicted probabilities by College and Gender are shown graphically in Fig. 5.6 (Panel C).

Discussion and Summary

This chapter provided an overview of two explanatory Rasch models: the Linear Logistic Rasch Model (LLRM) and the Latent Regression Rasch Model (LRRM). While traditional Rasch models focus on measurement, explanatory Rasch models incorporate item and person covariates to provide additional insights. The LLRM is an extension of the Rasch model that includes item-level covariates, while the LRRM includes person-level covariates. We illustrated these models using the Learning Stimulation Scale and the Attitude Toward Censorship (ATC) Scale.

The LLRM integrates item covariates into the Rasch framework to explain variations in item difficulty. This model can be estimated using GLMMs. GLMMs consist of three components: the random component (distribution of responses), the linking component (logit function), and the linear component (structural relationship between covariates and logits).

For dichotomous responses, we illustrated the LLRM using the Learning Stimulation Scale with items classified with respect to their focus on either child or adult activities. We used the eirm package for R to estimate parameters for the LLRM. Our key findings indicate that activities related to children are more frequently observed in home environments compared to adult-related activities. For polytomous responses, we illustrated the LLRM using the ATC Scale, which includes four response options (Strongly Disagree to Strongly Agree). Sentiment analysis was used to classify item valence (positive, negative, or neutral). The results suggest that items with positive valence were generally easier to endorse. However, item valence was not a statistically significant predictor of item location on the latent variable.

Explanatory Rasch models, such as the LRRM, incorporate person covariates into the Rasch model to examine their influence on individual abilities or attitudes. In this chapter, we extended our previous ATC Scale analysis by including education level and gender as person covariates. We estimated three LLRMs. The first LLRM included education level as a covariate. Our results indicated that college graduates showed higher support for censorship. The second LLRM included gender as a covariate. With this model, we observed that male respondents exhibited greater support for censorship compared to females. The third model included an interaction effect between education level and gender. No statistically significant interaction between education and gender was found with education level remaining the primary predictor of views toward censorship.

In summary, explanatory Rasch models provide deeper insights into item difficulty and person ability by incorporating covariates. The LLRM helps explain variations in item responses using item attributes, while the LRRM examines how personal characteristics influence response tendencies. These models enhance the interpretability and application of Rasch measurement models in educational and psychological assessments.

References

De Boeck, P., et al. (2011). The estimation of item response models with the lmer function from the lme4 package in R. *Journal of Statistical Software, 39*(12), 1–28.

De Boeck, P., & Wilson, M. R. (2016). Explanatory response models. In W.J. van der Linden (Ed.), Handbook of item response theory, Volume 1 (pp. 593–608). Chapman and Hall/CRC.

Engelhard, G., & Wind, S. A. (2018). *Invariant measurement with raters and rating scales: Rasch models for rater-mediated assessments.* Routledge.

Fischer, G. H. (1973). The linear logistic test model as an instrument in educational research. *Acta Psychologica, 3*, 359–374.

Jockers, M.L. (2015). Syuzhet: Extract Sentiment and Plot Arcs from Text. http://cran.r-project.org/web/packages/syuzhet/

Linacre, J. M. (1989). *Many-faceted Rasch measurement* (Doctoral dissertation, The University of Chicago).

Mohammad, S. M. (2016). Sentiment analysis: Detecting valence, emotions, and other affectual states from text. In H. L. Meiselman (Ed.), *Emotion measurement* (pp. 201–237). Woodhead Publishing.

Rosander, A. C., & Thurstone, L. L. (1931). Scale of attitude toward censorship: Scale no. 28. In L. L. Thurstone (Ed.), *The measurement of social attitudes*. University of Chicago Press.

Stanke, L., & Bulut, O. (2019). Explanatory item response models for polytomous item responses. *International Journal of Assessment Tools in Education, 6*(2), 259–278.

Tuerlinckx, F., & Wang, W. C. (2004). Models for polytomous data. In *Explanatory item response models: A generalized linear and nonlinear approach* (pp. 75–109). Springer.

Chapter 6
Rater-Mediated Assessments with Explanatory Rasch Models

> *... most of the reservations, regardless of how elegantly phrased, reflect fears that rating scale data are subjective (emphasizing, of course, the undesirable connotations of subjectivity), biased, and at worst, purposefully distorted. In the face of these often-warranted misgivings, it is not surprising that psychologists and other professionals who rely on rating data have devoted much time and effort to the development of techniques and procedures for assessing the veracity and psychometric qualities of their judgmental measures*
> (Saal et al., 1980, p. 413)

So far in this book, we have focused on *selected-response* items, where participants respond to items by selecting from a pre-specified list of response options. The person responses can be either dichotomous (e.g., incorrect, correct) or polytomous (e.g., strongly disagree, disagree, agree, and strongly agree). In this chapter, we focus on *rater-mediated assessments*. Rater-mediated assessments are measurement procedures in which raters engage in a judgmental procedure to score examinees' constructed responses or performances using a rating scale that represents a construct. Rater-mediated assessments are used in a variety of disciplinary areas and domains, such as writing assessments, music assessments, teacher evaluations, among others (Johnson et al., 2009).

Compared to selected-response assessments, rater-mediated assessments include several unique challenges related to rater judgment. Even when automated procedures are used to score performances (e.g., automated essay scoring), human rater judgment is required for some aspect of the scoring process, such as developing, evaluating, or calibrating the automated scoring process (Williamson et al., 2012). To the extent possible, measurement analyses for rater-mediated assessments aim to estimate examinee achievement such that these measures can be interpreted independently from the raters used to score performances. In this chapter, we refer to this idea as rater-invariant measurement.

In terms of measurement traditions (see Chapter 2), researchers who study rater-mediated assessments often use methods that reflect the Test Score Tradition (e.g., Generalizability) or the Scaling Tradition (e.g., Rasch models) to evaluate rater judgments and estimate examinee achievement. With test score approaches, researchers

G. Engelhard and S. A. Wind, *Invariant Measurement with Explanatory Rasch Models in the Human Sciences*, https://doi.org/10.1007/978-3-032-08816-1_6

often focus on evaluating rater reliability or rater agreement by comparing observed scores across raters and examinees. Within the scaling tradition, there is a rich body of literature in which researchers have considered how invariance principles can be extended to consider rater judgment. In this chapter, we consider how explanatory Rasch models provide a theoretically and practically useful framework in which to examine rater-mediated assessments. We consider how an explanatory Rasch modeling approach can be extended to consider and address unique challenges associated with rater-mediated assessments.

This chapter is organized as follows. In the next section, we describe an approach to modeling rater judgments using explanatory Rasch models. Then, we use an illustrative analysis of data from a rater-mediated writing assessment to demonstrate how this approach provides insight related to three special considerations for rater-mediated assessments: (1) data collection designs; (2) parameter interpretations; and (3) specific types of rater errors and systematic biases. We demonstrate the model specifications and special considerations using analyses of writing assessment data using the TAM package for R. We have integrated the corresponding R code with our descriptions, and the Appendix for this chapter includes all of the code used to conduct the analyses.

Explanatory Rasch Models for Rater-Mediated Assessments

Figure 6.1 presents the principles for invariant rater-mediated assessments. This figure is an extension of Fig. 2.8 in Chapter 2. The diagram demonstrates how rater judgments can be incorporated into an invariant measurement framework with an explanatory focus. As was true for the selected-response modeling applications that we have considered so far in this book, we emphasize invariance as a guiding principle for measurement with rater-mediated assessments, where measurement procedures reflect *rater judgments* of assessment elements. In these assessments, all aspects of measurement including constructs, persons, and items, must be extended to reflect the role of rater judgments. As shown in the figure, the construct is extended to a *rater-mediated construct* that reflects rater judgments. Likewise, person locations reflect rater interpretations of person performances or behaviors. Finally, item locations are extended to reflect rater judgments of assessment elements through which persons are evaluated, such as constructed response (CR) items or domains in an analytic scoring rubric. Together, these elements can be evaluated from an invariant measurement perspective.

Engelhard and Wind (2018) used a Rasch approach to consider invariant measurement with raters. They used the term "cues" to describe assessment components on which examinees receive ratings, such as CR items or domains in an analytic scoring rubric. They proposed the following guiding principles for invariant measurement with raters:

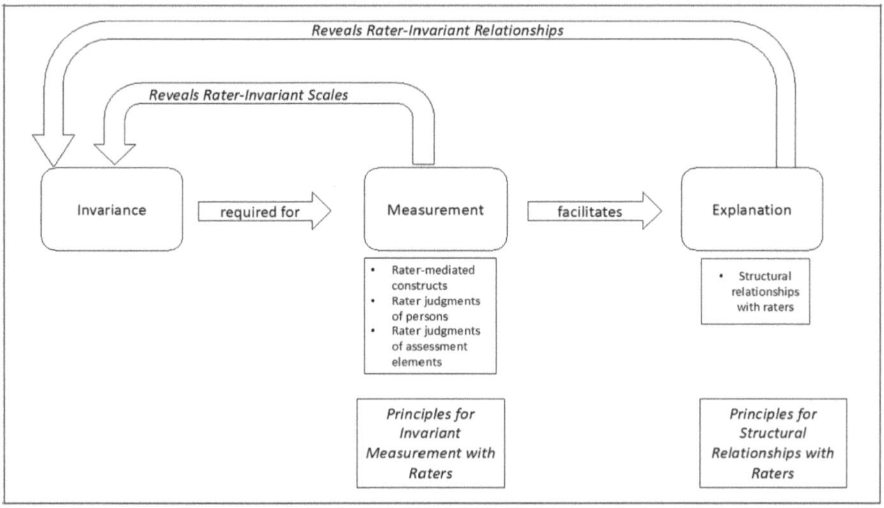

Fig. 6.1 Principles for Invariant Rater-Mediated Assessments

1. *Rater-invariant measurement of persons*: The measurement of persons must be independent of the particular raters that happen to be used in the assessment.
2. *Rater-invariant calibration of cues*: The calibration of the cues must be independent of the particular raters used in the assessment.
3. *Rater-invariant calibration of rating scales*: The structure of the rating categories must be independent of the particular raters used in the assessment.
4. *Invariant locations of raters*: The location of raters must be independent of the particular persons, cues, and rating scales used in the assessment.
5. *Rater-invariant Wright map*: Persons, cues, rating scales, and raters must be simultaneously located on an underlying latent continuum used in an assessment system.

Invariant measurement with raters ensures that the results from rater-mediated assessments can be interpreted independently from the individual raters, students, and components used in the assessment procedure. Engelhard and Wind (2018) demonstrated how evaluating rater-mediated assessments for adherence to these invariance principles is critical to ensure validity, reliability, and fairness in rater-mediated assessment systems.

Reflecting the focus of this book, invariant measurement with raters also facilitates explanatory analyses with which structural relationships can be explored. Compared to selected-response assessments, explanatory Rasch models are relatively common in research on rater-mediated assessments. Although it is not usually described as an explanatory Rasch model or included among discussions of explanatory IRT in general, Linacre's (1989) Many-Facet Rasch Model (MFRM) is an example of an explanatory Rasch model that is particularly useful in rater-mediated assessments. Linacre presented the MFRM to address practical concerns related to rater-mediated assessments, including the need to separate examinee achievement estimates from differences in individual rater judgments. Since then, researchers have used the MFRM to model and control for rater severity across a wide range of disciplinary areas including writing assessment (McNamara & Knoch, 2012), music performance assessment (Wesolowski & Wind, 2019), teacher evaluation (Wind & Jones, 2019a), standard setting (Kaliski et al., 2013), among others.

The MFRM is specified by extending a standard Rasch model (e.g., the Partial Credit Model) to include researcher-specified explanatory variables—called "facets". Facets can be related to items (e.g., item classifications), persons (e.g., person subgroups), or other aspects of a measurement context, such as raters. A general equation for the MFRM is:

$$\ln\left(\frac{P_{n(x=k)}}{P_{n(x=k-1)}}\right) = \theta_n - \sum_{facets} \varepsilon - \tau_k \tag{6.1}$$

where θ_n is the location of Person n on the latent variable, τ_k is the rating scale category threshold, which can be modified to reflect different standard Rasch models, and Σ_{facets} is a linear combination of researcher-specified facets. The linear combination of facets may include descriptive indicator variables (e.g., item and rater indicators) as well as explanatory variables (e.g., item or domain-related properties and person-related properties). When rater indicators are included in the MFRM, parameter estimates for the other facets are adjusted for differences in rater severity.

In Table 6.1, we propose a classification system for specifications of the MFRM that include different combinations of person, items/domains, and rater-related indicators and covariates. Connecting the MFRM with the language typically used with explanatory Rasch models, facets related to persons, items/domains, or rater characteristics can be viewed as a type of explanatory covariate. Descriptive versions of the MFRM can be specified that only include indicators, where the response probability is calculated using a combination of person indicators and indicators for explanatory facets that reflect an assessment system (e.g., raters and rubric domains). Alternatively, the MFRM may include some combination of indicators with covariates associated with person characteristics (e.g., examinee subgroups) or characteristics associated with explanatory facets (e.g., item classifications or rater characteristics). Various combinations of person and facet properties may be included to construct different types of explanatory MFRMs. We discuss some examples of these models in the paragraphs that follow.

Illustrative Data

To provide context for our discussion of MFRM specifications, we use illustrative data from a Georgia High School Writing Test that is a rater-mediated writing performance assessment for eighth grade students in the US. Our illustrative data come from a

Table 6.1 Descriptive and explanatory many-facet Rasch Models

Models		Person covariates	Domain /Item covariates	Rater covariates	Example equations (Logits)
Descriptive	MFRM-RS	No	No	No	$\ln\left(\frac{P_{nir(x=k)}}{P_{nir(x=k-1)}}\right) = \theta_n - \delta_\iota - \lambda_r - \tau_k,$
	MFRM-PC	No	No	No	$\ln\left(\frac{P_{nir(x=k)}}{P_{nir(x=k-1)}}\right) = \theta_n - \delta_\iota - \lambda_r - \tau_{rk}$
Explanatory	Person-Explanatory MFRM-RS	Yes	No	No	$\ln\left(\frac{P_{ngitr(x=k)}}{P_{ngitr(x=k-1)}}\right) = (\theta_n - \gamma_g) - \delta_\iota - \lambda_r - \tau_k,$
	Person-Explanatory MFRM-PC	Yes	No	No	$\ln\left(\frac{P_{ngitr(x=k)}}{P_{ngitr(x=k-1)}}\right) = (\theta_n - \gamma_g) - \delta_\iota - \lambda_r - \tau_{gk},$
	Person-Explanatory MFRM with interactions (RS or PC)	Yes	No	No	$\ln\left(\frac{P_{ngir(x=k)}}{P_{ngir(x=k-1)}}\right) = (\theta_n - \gamma_g) - \delta_\iota - (\lambda_r - \lambda_r\gamma_g) - \tau_k.$
	Domain/ Item-Explanatory MFRM (RS or PC)	No	Yes	No	$\ln\left(\frac{P_{nitr(x=k)}}{P_{nitr(x=k-1)}}\right) = \theta_n - (\delta_\iota - \mu_t) - \lambda_r - \tau_k,$
	Rater-Explanatory MFRM (RS or PC)	No	No	Yes	$\ln\left(\frac{P_{nirl(x=k)}}{P_{nirl(x=k-1)}}\right) = \theta_n - \delta_\iota - (\lambda_r - \beta_l) - \tau_k,$
	Fully-Explanatory MFRM (RS or PC)	Yes	Yes	Yes	$\ln\left(\frac{P_{ngitr(x=k)}}{P_{ngitr(x=k-1)}}\right) = (\theta_n - \gamma_g) - (\delta_\iota - \mu_t) - (\lambda_r - \beta_l) - \tau_k,$

Note Model parameters are represented as follows: θ = person locations; δ = domain locations; λ = rater locations; τ = threshold locations; γ = person-related covariates; β = domain-related covariates

sample of 365 students who wrote persuasive essays as part of this assessment. A group of 21 raters scored each student's essay using a four-category rating scale in which higher ratings indicated higher levels of writing proficiency; for our analysis, we recoded the scale to range from 0 to 3. Each point value represents a rating between one and four, with a score of one as "inadequate," two as "poor," three as "good," and four as "very good." The raters scored each student's essay using an analytic rubric with four domains: Conventions, Organization, Sentence Formation, and Style. All raters scored all students on all domains.

We analyzed the writing assessment data with various specifications of the MFRM using the TAM package for R (Robitzsch et al., 2020) as the main analytic tool. We also used functions from the psych package (Revelle, 2016) and WrightMap package (Torres Irribarra & Freund, 2014). After loading the required packages and setting the working directory to the location in which we stored the data file, we imported the data. The data file is structured such that each row includes a single student's ratings from all 21 raters on a single domain. Reflecting the four domains in the analytic rubric, there are four rows associated with each student.

```
## Import the writing assessment data:
writing.all <- read.csv("GA_writing_wide_format.csv")
```

Before we applied the MFRM analyses, we loaded a custom function with which to calculate the reliability of separation statistic for individual facets:

```
## Load a custom function for separation reliability:
facet.sep.rel <- function(location.estimates, location.se){
OV <- var(location.estimates)
EV <- mean(location.se^2)
sep.rel <- (OV—EV)/OV
print(paste("sep.rel=", round(sep.rel, digits = 2)))
}
```

Descriptive MFRM

Our first example is a descriptive MFRM that could be used with a rater- mediated performance assessment in which raters score student performances using an analytic rubric with domains. The model includes indicators for students, raters, and domains, but no specific explanatory properties are included. A descriptive MFRM model could be stated as:

$$\ln\left(\frac{P_{nir(x=k)}}{P_{nir(x=k-1)}}\right) = \theta_n - \delta_\iota - \lambda_r - \tau_k \tag{6.2}$$

where $_n$ is the location of Person n on the latent variable (student achievement), δ_i is the location of domain i on the latent variable (domain difficulty), λ_r is the location of Rater r on the latent variable (rater severity), and τ_k is the location of rating scale threshold k. Equation 6.2 is a rating scale (Andrich, 2018) formulation of the MFRM (i.e., MFRM-RS). In this model specification, raters and items are facets related to student ratings. Assuming adequate model-data fit, student location and item difficulty parameters can be adjusted for differences in rater severity.

To apply Equation 6.2 in the TAM package (Robitzsch et al., 2020), we need to specify the model components in individual objects for reference in the estimation function. We started by identifying the matrix of responses for analysis. By default in the TAM functions for the MFRM, individual columns in the response matrix are labeled as "items", even if they actually represent other facet elements, such as raters or domains. With this in mind, we extracted the response matrix with rater judgments associated with individual students on each domain and stored it in a data frame object called "ratings.df":

```
# response matrix (raters are columns; labeled as "items" by
default in TAM)
ratings <- subset(writing.all, select = c(rater_1 : rater_
21))
ratings.df <- as.data.frame(ratings)
names(ratings.df) <- c(1:21)
```

Then, we re-scaled the responses such that the lowest category was set to 0:

```
## rescale to start at zero:
ratings.df.zero <- ratings.df - 1
```

Next, we saved the descriptive facet in a data frame object labeled "facets." For this model specification, we are using domain as the single descriptive facet:

```
## identify the facets (domain)
facets <- writing.all[ , "domain", drop = FALSE]
names(facets) <- c("domain")
```

Next, we identified the examinee indicators in an object called "students":

```
## identify the examinee indicators (student ids)
students <- writing.all$student.id
```

The final step in preparing for the MFRM analysis is to specify the equation. In TAM, MFRM equations with the RS formulation are specified using the following general form: [model name] <- ~ item + [facet names] + step. Recall that by default, elements represented in columns of the response matrix are always labeled "items."

Accordingly, we specified the equation as follows, recognizing that the label "item" actually refers to raters in this case:

```
## specify the MFRM equation ("item" refers to raters)
RS_MFRM <- ~ item + domain + step
```

Finally, we estimated the model using the tam.mml.mfr() function with the following specifications to reflect our response matrix, facets, and equation:

```
# Run the model
RS_MFR_model <- tam.mml.mfr(resp = ratings.df.zero, facets =
facets, formulaA = RS_MFRM, pid = students, verbose = FALSE,
constraint = "items")
```

The code in the Appendix includes additional analyses based on Equation 6.2, including extracting estimates for individual facets and evaluating model-data fit. We discuss these results later in the chapter.

As an alternative to the RS formulation of the model, a descriptive MFRM could also be specified using a Partial Credit (PC; Masters, 1982) model formulation. Researchers often examine polytomous ratings for evidence of adequate rating scale functioning using the PCM. In a rater-mediated assessment context, PC formulations of the MFRM can provide insight into rating scale functioning related to other facets such as raters or items. For example, we can examine individual raters' use of the rating scale using rater-specific thresholds with the following descriptive MFRM-PC:

$$\ln\left(\frac{P_{nir(x=k)}}{P_{nir(x=k-1)}}\right) = \theta_n - \delta_\iota - \lambda_r - \tau_{rk} \tag{6.3}$$

where all of the parameters are defined as before, and τ_{rk} is the rater-specific threshold parameter. With this model, we can examine rating scale functioning specific to individual raters, including threshold ordering and precision.

To estimate the model shown in Equation 6.3 with TAM, we follow the same preparatory steps as discussed for Equation 6.2 with the exception of the equation specification. To specify a PC formulation of the model, we modify the equation object with "item:step" to indicate rater-specific threshold estimates:

```
## specify the MFRM in an object
PC_MFRM <- ~ item + domain + item:step
```

As a third alternative, we could also specify a descriptive MFRM-PC to examine rating scale functioning as it relates to domains:

$$\ln\left(\frac{P_{nir(x=k)}}{P_{nir(x=k-1)}}\right) = \theta_n - \delta_\iota - \lambda_r - \tau_{ik} \tag{6.4}$$

where τ_{ik} is the domain-specific threshold parameter.

There are several ways in which we could estimate Equation 6.4 in TAM. To present a straightforward illustration, we used a re-arranged long-format version of the writing assessment data in which the columns in the response matrix represent domains. Each student appears in 21 rows that reflect each of the 21 raters' scores. We imported the updated data file using read.csv() and sorted it by student id:

```
# import the long-format version of the data:
writing <- read.csv("writing_long_domains.csv")
# With long format data, we need to ensure that the person
identification numbers
# (in this case, student ids) are sorted from low to high before
we can run the analysis.
writing <- writing[order(writing$student),]
```

With this data structure, the facet labeled "items" by default in TAM refers to domains. We specified the components of the model by identifying the facets (raters), response matrix, and student ids:

```
## identify the facets (raters)
writing.facets <- writing[, c("rater"), drop = FALSE]
## identify the examinee indicators (student ids)
writing.pid <- writing$student
## identify the response matrix
writing.resp <- subset(writing, select = -c(student, gender,
rater))
```

Finally, we specified the model equation with the PC formulation indicated using "item:step":

```
## specify the MFRM equation ("item" refers to domains)
PC.writing.formula <- ~ item + rater + item:step
```

We estimated the model using the following code:

```
## run the PC-MFRM model
```

```
domain_PC_MFRM.model    <-    tam.mml.mfr(resp=writing.resp,
facets=writing.facets,         formulaA=PC.writing.formula,
pid=writing.pid,verbose = FALSE, constraint = "items")
```

We return to this model to consider results later in the chapter.

Explanatory MFRM

Turning now to explanatory MFRMs, additional facets can be added to a MFRM-RS or MFRM-PC that reflect explanatory hypotheses related to person properties (e.g., person subgroups). For example, researchers may be interested in modeling the effects of person subgroups in a rater-mediated assessment using the following person-explanatory MFRM-RS:

$$\ln\left(\frac{P_{ngitr(x=k)}}{P_{ngitr(x=k-1)}}\right) = (\theta_n - \gamma_g) - \delta_\iota - \lambda_r - \tau_k. \tag{6.5}$$

In Equation 6.5, $_{n,}$ $\delta_{i,}$ $\lambda_{r,}$ and τ_k are defined as in Equation 6.2. The model also includes a student subgroup facet (γ_g), which is a person-explanatory variable. The student subgroup facet describes the location of student subgroups on the latent variable (e.g., achievement within demographic groups).

We can specify this model in TAM using an adapted version of our code related to Equation 6.5. We will use the wide format version of the writing assessment data (named "writing.all").

```
## Import the writing assessment data:
writing.all <- read.csv("GA_writing_wide_format.csv")
```

As before, after importing the data, we identify the response matrix, where columns represent individual raters. We re-scale the responses such that the lowest response category equals zero:

```
# identify the response matrix (raters are columns; labeled as
"items" by default in TAM)
ratings <- subset(writing.all, select = c(rater_1 : rater_
21))
ratings.df <- as.data.frame(ratings)
names(ratings.df) <- c(1:21)
## rescale to start at zero:
ratings.df.zero <- ratings.df - 1
```

Then, we identify the facets (student gender and domain) and examinee indicators. For generality, we refer to the gender facet as "subgroup" in this code:

```
## identify the facets (gender, domain)
facets <- writing.all[ , c("gender", "domain"), drop = FALSE]
names(facets) <- c("subgroup", "domain")
## identify the examinee indicators (student ids)
students <- writing.all$student.id
```

We specify the equation and estimate the model as follows:

```
## specify the MFRM equation ("item" refers to raters)
RS_MFRM <- ~ item + subgroup + domain + item*subgroup + step
## Run the model
RS_MFR_model <- tam.mml.mfr(resp = ratings.df.zero, facets =
facets, formulaA = RS_MFRM, pid = students, verbose = FALSE,
constraint = "items")
```

We return to this model to consider results later in the chapter.

Similarly, the person-explanatory MFRM could be specified using a PCM formulation in order to examine differences in rating scale category use between student subgroups:

$$\ln\left(\frac{P_{ngitr(x=k)}}{P_{ngitr(x=k-1)}}\right) = \left(\theta_n - \gamma_g\right) - \delta_\iota - \lambda_r - \tau_{gk} \tag{6.6}$$

Code related to this model is included in the supplementary material for Chapter 6.

Another common use of the MFRM is to explore interactions between facets. In the context of a rater-mediated assessment, researchers may be interested in identifying individual raters who exercise different levels of severity between student subgroups using a person-explanatory MFRM-RS model such as:

$$\ln\left(\frac{P_{ngir(x=k)}}{P_{ngir(x=k-1)}}\right) = \left(\theta_n - \gamma_g\right) - \delta_\iota - \left(\lambda_r - \lambda_r\gamma_g\right) - \tau_k \tag{6.7}$$

In Equation 6.7, $\lambda_r\gamma_g$ is the interaction between rater severity and student subgroup classifications. This facet provides insight into the degree to which rater severity is invariant over student subgroups. In theory, interactions could be added between any of the explanatory facets to test hypotheses related to invariance. Code related to this model is included in the supplementary material for Chapter 6. We revisit the idea of interaction effects with raters later in this chapter.

It is also possible to develop domain or item-explanatory MFRMs. Researchers may be interested in modeling the properties of items/domains. For example, a domain-explanatory MFRM-RS or MFRM-PC could be used in a rater-mediated assessment in which the domains in an analytic rubric were classified to reflect different categories (e.g., meaning-related or mechanics-related domains for a writing assessment). Using the MFRM-RS formulation, a domain-explanatory MFRM-RS might be specified as:

$$\ln\left(\frac{P_{nitr(x=k)}}{P_{nitr(x=k-1)}}\right) = \theta_n - (\delta_\iota - \mu_t) - \lambda_r - \tau_k \tag{6.8}$$

where all of the parameters are defined as before and μ_t is a domain-explanatory facet that reflects domain classifications. This model could also be modified to reflect a PC specification (domain/item-explanatory MFRM-PC) or to include interaction terms.

Researchers may also be interested in examining the effects of rater background characteristics such as level of rating experience, language background, or training procedure. A rater-explanatory MFRM can be used to examine the effects of these characteristics using either a RS or PC model formulation. For example, the following MFRM-RS could be used to examine the explanatory effects of rater language background in a rater-mediated writing assessment:

$$\ln\left(\frac{P_{nirl(x=k)}}{P_{nirl(x=k-1)}}\right) = \theta_n - \delta_\iota - (\lambda_r - \beta_l) - \tau_k \tag{6.9}$$

where all of the parameters are defined as before and β_l is a rater-explanatory facet that reflects raters' classification within language background subgroups. This model could also be modified to reflect a PC model specification (rater-explanatory MFRM-PC) or to include interaction terms.

Finally, combining the ideas from the previous explanatory MFRM specifications, a fully-explanatory MFRM-RS or MFRM-PC could be specified that includes properties associated with persons, domains/items, and raters. For example, student subgroups, domain classifications, and rater characteristics could be explored using the following MFRM-RS:

$$\ln\left(\frac{P_{ngitr(x=k)}}{P_{ngitr(x=k-1)}}\right) = \left(\theta_n - \gamma_g\right) - (\delta_\iota - \mu_t) - (\lambda_r - \beta_l) - \tau_k \tag{6.10}$$

where all of the parameters are defined as before. This model could be modified to reflect a MFRM-PC specification or to include interaction terms associated with any combination of facets.

Special Considerations for Measurement and Explanation in Rater-Mediated Assessments

In this section, we use an illustrative analysis of data from a rater-mediated writing assessment to demonstrate the use of the MFRM as an explanatory Rasch model. We organize our discussion around several considerations that are central to the design and use of measurement models in rater-mediated assessments:

1. data collection designs;
2. parameter interpretations;
3. model-data fit for explanatory Rasch models with raters; and
4. specific types of rater errors and biases.

We use illustrative data from a Georgia High School Writing Test described earlier in this chapter. In the following sections, we use the writing data to discuss and illustrate analyses related to the use of explanatory Rasch models with rater-mediated performance assessments.

Data Collection Designs for Rater-Mediated Assessments

Compared to selected-response assessments, data collection designs (i.e., scoring designs) for rater-mediated assessments are often complex and resource-intensive—requiring substantial time and other resources to obtain enough scores for examinee performances to facilitate a valid, reliable, and fair interpretation and use of assessment results. Practical constraints in most performance assessment systems preclude *complete scoring designs* in which every rater scores every examinee on every assessment component (e.g., CR item or rubric domain). More typically, a small subset of raters from a larger rater pool typically scores each performance—resulting in an *incomplete scoring design.* When incomplete designs are used, it is necessary to ensure that student achievement can be interpreted separately from rater severity. In other words, we need to ensure that student achievement estimates are comparable across different raters.

One way to facilitate comparisons in incomplete scoring designs is to incorporate connections between components of the assessment procedure. When sufficient connections are present, such as raters scoring students in common with other raters, scaling models such as the MFRM can provide comparable parameter estimates in incomplete scoring designs. In previous studies, several researchers have discussed the flexibility of the MFRM for parameter estimation with various types of incomplete scoring designs, such as those that may be used in rater-mediated performance assessments (Engelhard, 1997; Schumacker, 1999). These incomplete design specifications reflect experimental design principles with balanced and incomplete block designs (Kirk, 1995), as well as ideas from test equating with common items or persons (Wolfe, 2004).

We consider three major types of scoring designs for rater-mediated assessments that facilitate analyses with explanatory Rasch models such as the MFRM: (1) complete designs, (2) linked designs, and (3) anchor designs. Figure 6.2 illustrates these three designs, and we discuss each of them below.

In complete scoring designs for rater-mediated assessments, every rater scores every examinee on every assessment component (e.g., CR item or rubric domain). Although complete designs are rare in operational assessment programs, they may be used during assessment development, rater training, or rater evaluation procedures when it is especially important to gather detailed information with which to evaluate measurement quality. Our illustrative writing assessment dataset is an example of a complete scoring design because each of the raters scored each of the students on all of the assessment domains.

Figure 6.2A illustrates a complete scoring design for a rater-mediated assessment using a matrix in which the rows represent student performances and the columns

Scoring Design	**Ratings on Assessment Components**						
A. Complete Scoring Design	**Student Performance Number**	**Rater Number**					
		1	**2**	**3**	**4**	**…**	***i***
	1	X	X	X	X	…	X
	2	X	X	X	X	…	X
	3	X	X	X	X	…	X
	4	X	X	X	X	…	X
	…	…	…	…	…	…	X
	n	X	X	X	X	…	X
B. Linked Design	**Student Performance Number**	**Rater Number**					
		1	2	3	4	…	*i*
	1	X	X				
	2		X	X			
	3			X	X		
	4				X	…	
	…					…	
	n	X					X
C. Anchor Design	**Student Performance Number**	**Rater Number**					
		1	2	3	4	…	*i*
	Anchor Performance 1	X	X	X	X	…	X
	Anchor Performance 2	X	X	X	X	…	X
	Anchor Performance 3	X	X	X	X	…	X
	1	X					
	2		X				
	3			X			
	4				X	…	
	…					…	
	n						X

Fig. 6.2 Illustrations of scoring designs for rater-mediated assessments

represent raters. Cells marked with an "X" indicate that the rater shown in the column scored the performance shown in the row on all assessment components.

A major advantage of complete scoring designs is that differences in rater severity, as well as differences in rating quality (e.g., the presence of rater effects or rater misfit) impact all examinees in the same way. This common impact of rater-related differences facilitates comparisons between examinees. However, even with complete designs, a measurement modeling approach is still useful because student achievement estimates are adjusted to reflect variations in rater judgment across the rater sample such that student achievement estimates reflect the overall average level of rater severity. Because differences in severity persist even after extensive rater training (Knoch et al., 2007; Lumley & McNamara, 1995; Raczynski et al., 2015), these model-based achievement estimates facilitate rater-invariant interpretations of student achievement.

When linked scoring designs are used, examinee performances receive scores from a subset of raters from the larger rater pool, and raters are linked to one another through common examinee performances or other assessment components (e.g., CR items). A variety of linked scoring designs for rater-mediated assessments appear throughout the literature, with differences in the number of raters who score each performance and procedures for assigning raters to performances.

For example, in the linked design shown in Fig. 6.2B, Rater 2 scored performances in common with Rater 1 and Rater 3. Likewise, Rater 3 scored performances in common with Rater 2 and Rater 4. The systematic connections between raters facilitate the estimation of rater severity, student achievement, and other parameters using explanatory Rasch models such as the MFRM (Engelhard, 1997; Schumacker, 1999). Other, more-complex designs for linking raters such as random rater assignment or spiral designs may be used depending on the nature of the assessment and scoring procedures (Hombo et al., 2001; Myford & Wolfe, 2000).

Anchor scoring designs for rater-mediated assessments include an "anchor set" of examinee performances that are scored by all raters. Anchor designs may be paired with a variety of incomplete scoring designs as a method for strengthening connections between raters, including various types of linked designs or disconnected designs that do not include systematic links between raters.

For example, the anchor design in Fig. 6.2C includes three anchor performances that were scored by all raters—reflecting a complete scoring design for that subset of performances. These common observations provide information with which to link raters across other performances in the operational sample. However, there are no connections between raters or students outside of the anchor set, because only one rater scored each performance, and raters did not score any performances in common with any other raters outside of the anchor set. In this design, the anchor performances connect the otherwise disconnected raters such that parameter estimates can be compared across student performances and raters.

Other variations on anchor designs include using a single common rater to score all examinee performances, including anchor performances, to increase connections in linked designs, and using an external anchor, such as a set of multiple-choice (MC) items to connect students when it is not possible to incorporate systematic links in the scoring design.

Researchers have considered several issues related to the use of anchor designs in rater-mediated assessments, including the minimum size of linking sets and the effects of different achievement levels, score distributions, and measurement characteristics (e.g., model-data fit) within the linking set. In general, results from these studies suggest that it is possible to identify rater effects in very sparse rating designs as long as connectivity is established (Jones & Wind, 2018; Wind & Ge, 2021; Wind & Jones, 2017, 2018, 2019b).

Interpreting Explanatory Rasch Model Parameters in Rater-Mediated Assessments

The next special consideration with rater-mediated assessments is related to the interpretation of parameters in MFRMs. After data are collected from a rater-mediated assessment, explanatory Rasch models such as the MFRM can be used to estimate parameters for raters, examinees, and other assessment components. Assuming sufficient connectivity in the scoring design and adequate model-data fit, these parameters can generally be interpreted as the locations of the assessment components on a linear scale that represents the rater-mediated construct. Moreover, researchers can display parameter estimates from explanatory Rasch models on a common metric using a rater-mediated Wright Map as a visual summary of the results.

In this section, we explore and interpret rater-mediated Wright Maps from analyses with the illustrative data to demonstrate some special considerations related to parameter interpretation for explanatory Rasch models with raters. We estimated each model and completed all related analyses using TAM (Robitzsch et al., 2020). We provide more details about the R code and analysis for the first model (Equation 6.2) and refer interested readers to the Appendix for our annotated code with full analyses related to the other models.

We will begin our consideration of these ideas using results from our analysis based on Equation 6.2, which is a descriptive MFRM-RS. Recall that we prepared the writing assessment data and applied the model earlier in this chapter using the tam.mml.mfr() function. After estimating the model, we extracted location estimates from the model object for the domain and rater facets. We also applied our custom function to calculate reliability of separation for these facets.

First, we examine the rater location estimates using the following code.

```
## Extract location estimates specific to each facet:
facet.estimates <- RS_MFR_model$xsi.facets
### Extract rater estimates:
```

```
rater.results <- subset(facet.estimates,
facet.estimates$facet == "item")
rater.results$rater.id <- as.numeric(rater.results$parameter)
View(rater.results)
```

For raters, the overall location estimates for the raters reflect their level of severity across students and domains. In this analysis, rater severity locations ranged from $\lambda = -0.55$ logits ($SE = 0.04$) for Rater 15, who was the most lenient rater, to 0.75 logits ($SE = 0.04$) for Rater 9, who was the most severe rater. We calculated the reliability of separation statistic for raters with our custom function:

```
### Calculate rater reliability of separation:
facet.sep.rel(location.estimates = rater.results$xsi,
location.se = rater.results$se.xsi)
```

For raters, the reliability of separation statistic was equal to 0.98, which indicates distinct locations on the rater-mediated construct for individual raters.

Next, we examined the location estimates, standard errors, and reliability of separation for the domain facet.

```
### Extract domain estimates:
domain.results <- subset(facet.estimates,
facet.estimates$facet == "domain")
View(domain.results)
### Calculate domain reliability of separation :
facet.sep.rel(location.estimates = domain.results$xsi,
location.se = domain.results$se.xsi)
```

Domain location estimates ranged from $-0.89 \leq \delta \leq 0.66$. These location estimates reflect rater judgments of domain difficulty, where Sentence Formation had the lowest location ($\delta = -0.89$)—indicating that raters judged this domain to be easiest and tended to assign higher ratings, followed by Conventions ($\delta = -0.08$), Style ($\delta =$ 031), and Organization ($\delta = 0.66$). The reliability of separation statistic for domains indicated high reliability (> 0.99), suggesting that the estimated domain locations on the rater-mediated construct were distinct.

Finally, we extracted location estimates for the thresholds, which are labeled as a facet by default in TAM.

```
threshold.results <- subset(facet.estimates,
facet.estimates$facet == "step")
View(threshold.results)
```

Because the analysis is based on a RS formulation of the model, the relative distance between adjacent thresholds is the same for all raters. For the four-category ordinal scale, the threshold locations were equal to τ_1 = -3.53, τ_2 = 0.07, and τ_3 = 3.46. These threshold estimates reflect raters' judgments of the difficulty associated with the rating scale categories. In this analysis, the thresholds were ordered as expected and distinct, such that the rating scale categories reflected increasing levels of judged writing achievement as categories progressed from low to high.

To facilitate construction of our WrightMap based on this model, we organized the threshold estimates into a matrix with values specific to each rater using a for-loop. Values in the matrix reflect the combination of each rater's overall severity with threshold locations on the logit scale.

```
### Organize the threshold estimates into a matrix for indi-
vidual raters:
rater_thresholds    <-    matrix(data    =    NA,    nrow    =
nrow(rater.results), ncol = nrow(threshold.results))
for(rater in 1:nrow(rater.results)){
for(tau in 1:nrow(threshold.results)){
rater_thresholds[rater,tau] <- (rater.results$xsi[rater] +
threshold.results$xsi[tau])
}
}
View(rater_thresholds)
```

To examine results related to students, it is necessary to estimate student locations using the model object and the tam.wle() function. The following code estimates student locations and organizes them into a data frame object along with the id variable and standard error. Then, we used summary statistics and calculated the reliability of separation statistic for students to examine the results in more detail.

```
## Estimate student locations:
student.ach <- tam.wle(RS_MFR_model)
### Store the student identification numbers, location esti-
mates, and standard errors in a new object
student.locations_RSMFR <- cbind.data.frame(student.ach$pid,
student.ach$theta, student.ach$error)
### Name the columns in the data.frame:
names(student.locations_RSMFR) <- c("id", "theta", "se")
## Request summary statistics:
describe(student.locations_RSMFR)
## Calculate reliability of separation for students:
facet.sep.rel(location.estimates    =    student.locations_
RSMFR$theta,
location.se = student.locations_RSMFR$se)
```

For this analysis, estimates of student locations reflect rater judgments of student writing achievement based on the analytic scoring rubric. Students with higher locations were judged to have higher levels of writing proficiency, and students with lower locations were judged to have lower levels of writing proficiency. Student location estimates ranged from $\theta = -7.25$ for the student with the lowest judged level of writing achievement to $\theta = 7.68$ for the student with the highest judged level of achievement. The average student location was equal to $\theta = 0.81$ logits. Standard errors for the student achievement estimates ranged from $0.20 \leq SE \leq 0.83$. The reliability of separation statistic indicated precise distinctions between location estimates for individual students: $rel_\theta = 0.99$. Assuming adequate model-data fit (discussed further below), these student location estimates are adjusted for differences in rater severity and domain difficulty.

Figure 6.3 summarizes the results from our analysis of the writing assessment data using Equation 6.2. We generated the Wright Map based on this model using the following code. We modified the default code for the WrightMap() function to create a custom display that includes the domain facet as well as both overall rater severity estimates and threshold locations. This required suppressing some warnings and overlaying two versions of the figure.

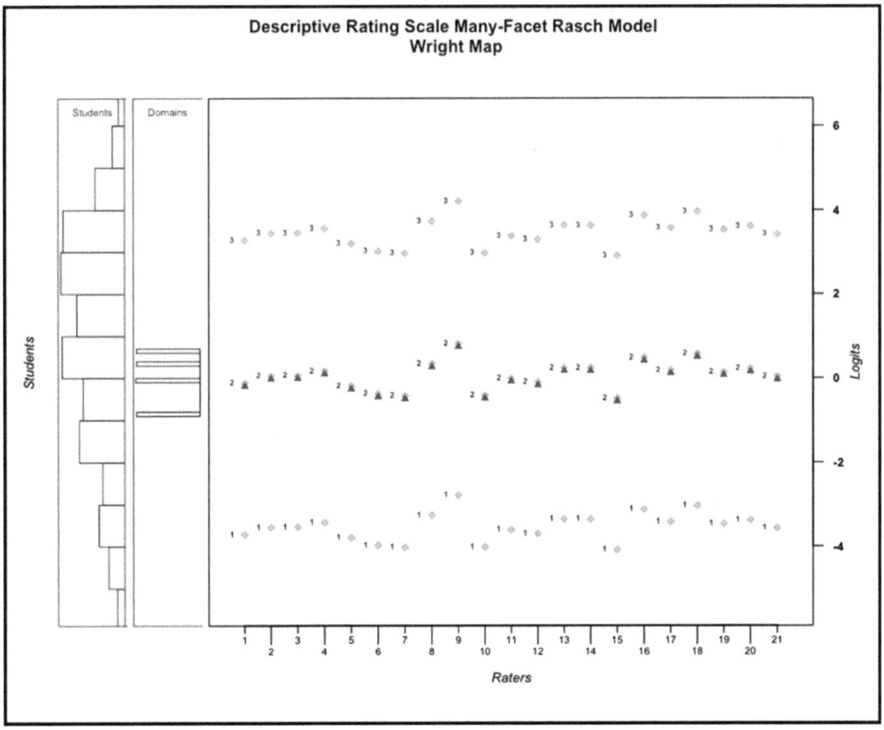

Fig. 6.3 Rater-mediated wright map for a descriptive RS-MFRM

```
## plot the Wright Map
graphics.off()
#* Note: We have suppressed a warning message here
#* that occurs due to the way we plotted the domain facet.
#* No need to worry about the warning.
suppressWarnings(wrightMap(thetas = cbind(student.locations_
RSMFR$theta, domain.results$xsi),
axis.persons = "Students",
dim.names = c("Students", "Domains"),
thresholds = rater_thresholds,
show.thr.lab = TRUE,
thr.lab.pos = 2,
label.items.rows= 2,
label.items = rater.results$parameter,
axis.items = "Raters",
main.title = "Descriptive Rating Scale Many-Facet Rasch Model
\nWright Map",
cex.main = .6,
yrange = c(-6, 6)))
par(new = T)
suppressWarnings(wrightMap(thetas = cbind(student.locations_
RSMFR$theta, domain.results$xsi),
axis.persons = "Students",
dim.names = c("Students", "Domains"),
thresholds = rater.results$xsi,
show.thr.lab = FALSE,
label.items.rows= 2,
label.items = rater.results$parameter,
axis.items = "Raters",
main.title = "",
cex.main = .6,
yrange = c(-6, 6),
thr.sym.pch = 17,
thr.sym.lwd = 2,
thr.sym.col.fg = "blue",
thr.sym.col.bg = "blue"))
```

We refer to Fig. 6.3 as a *rater-mediated Wright Map* to emphasize the central role of rater judgment in rater-mediated assessments. The units on the right vertical axis show the log-odds (logit) scale on which all of the facets in the model are estimated. This scale reflects the rater-mediated writing achievement construct. The left-most column displays a histogram of student achievement parameters. The second-from-the-left column shows a histogram of domain location estimates. Finally, the large central panel shows location estimates and rating scale category threshold estimates for each rater. The light grey diamond-shaped plotting symbols are the threshold estimates, and the darker triangle symbols show the overall location estimates for individual raters.

Returning to our discussion of alternative specifications for the MFRM in Section 1 of this chapter, Fig. 6.3, 6.6, 6.7 6.8 show rater-mediated Wright Maps based on analyses with the models reflected in Equations 6.3 through 6.5. The R code in the Appendix for this chapter includes detailed analyses related to each of these models used to generate the Wright Map displays. We provide a brief description of the Wright Maps here.

Figure 6.6 is a rater-mediated Wright Map that corresponds to Equation 6.3, in which the rating scale category thresholds are calculated specific to each rater using the MFRM-PC. This model specification allows us to explore rater-specific differences in rating scale interpretation and use. Although there were some differences in the relative distance between thresholds, the rating scale category thresholds were ordered as expected and distinct for all raters.

Next, descriptive MFRM-PC with Domain-Specific Thresholds can be estimated and examined. Figure 6.7 shows a rater-mediated Wright Map that corresponds to Equation 6.4, where the rating scale category thresholds are calculated specific to domains from the analytic scoring rubric. This model specification allows us to consider the degree to which the overall group of raters interprets the rating scale categories in a similar way across rubric domains.

Finally, it is interesting to explore a person-explanatory MFRM-RS. Figure 6.7 is a rater-mediated Wright Map that reflects the person-explanatory MFRM-RS given in Equation 6.5, in which student gender subgroups are added as a person- (student) explanatory facet. This version of the Wright Map includes location estimates for the student gender subgroups in a histogram. With this model, the estimated locations for the gender subgroups were as follows for male students = –0.60 ($SE = 0.01$) and female students = 0.60 ($SE = 0.01$), with a separation reliability > 0.99—suggesting that there were discernable differences in rater judgments of student achievement between subgroups.

Model-Data Fit for Explanatory Rasch Models with Raters

Evidence of adequate model-data fit is necessary to support interpretation of the rater-mediated Wright Map. For the current analysis with the MFRM, we will focus on element-level fit based on residuals associated with individual students, domains, and raters.

When a MFRM approach is used, it is possible to examine residual-based fit statistics for individual facets in a similar fashion to the item- and person-level fit statistics that are typically used with standard Rasch models. Infit mean square error (*MSE*) and outfit *MSE* statistics can be calculated using standardized residuals associated with individual elements within explanatory facets, such as individual raters or domains. Accordingly, researchers can examine and evaluate model-data fit in detail for explanatory variables using the same procedures as are typically used with standard models. This detailed fit analysis is a practical advantage of using a MFRM approach to explanatory Rasch modeling that facilitates in-depth examination, understanding, and in some cases, improvement of a measurement procedure.

First, we calculated fit statistics for students using the tam.personfit() function. Then, we calculated summary statistics for the fit results.

```
## Student fit
# Examine student fit using numeric infit and outfit statistics
student.fit <- tam.personfit(RS_MFR_model)
describe(student.fit)
```

On average, the person fit *MSE* statistics were close to 1.00, suggesting overall adequate fit, with some variation for individual students.

In TAM analyses with the MFRM, facet-related *MSE* fit statistics are organized using combinations of the item facet (in this case, raters) with levels of the descriptive facet (domains). In our example, *MSE* statistics are calculated for each rater specific to each domain. After calculating the fit statistics, we organized the results into a matrix such that we could consider infit and outfit *MSE* values related to individual raters. This process required some manipulation to account for the specific number of domains in our analysis.

```
## Rater Fit
# Examine model-data fit related to the domain and rater facets
rater.fit.all <- msq.itemfit(RS_MFR_model)
rater.domain.fit <- as.data.frame(rater.fit.all$itemfit)
# Examine fit statistics as they apply to individual raters
ndomains <- nrow(domain.results)
rater.fit <- matrix(data = NA, nrow = ncol(ratings), ncol =
(ndomains * 4) + 1 )
for(rater.number in 1:ncol(ratings)){
# calculate rater-specific fit statistics:
rater.outfit <- rater.domain.fit$Outfit[((rater.number*ndomains)−
(ndomains−1)) : (rater.number*ndomains)]
rater.infit <- rater.domain.fit$Infit[((rater.number*ndomains)−
(ndomains−1)) : (rater.number*ndomains)]
rater.std.outfit <- rater.domain.fit$Outfit_
t[((rater.number*ndomains)−(ndomains−1)) :
(rater.number*ndomains)]
rater.std.infit <- rater.domain.fit$Infit_
t[((rater.number*ndomains)−(ndomains−1)) :
(rater.number*ndomains)]
# add the fit statistics to the matrix:
rater.fit[rater.number, ] <- c(rater.number, rater.outfit,
rater.infit,
rater.std.outfit, rater.std.infit)
# Convert the rater fit results to a dataframe object and add mean-
ingful column names:
rater.fit_results <- as.data.frame(rater.fit)
infit_mse_labels <- NULL
for(domain in 1:ndomains){
```

```
infit_mse_labels[domain] <- paste("Infit_MSE_domain", domain, sep
= "")
}
outfit_mse_labels <- NULL
for(domain in 1:ndomains){
outfit_mse_labels[domain] <- paste("Outfit_MSE_domain", domain,
sep = "")
}
std_infit_mse_labels <- NULL
for(domain in 1:ndomains){
std_infit_mse_labels[domain]  <-  paste("Std.Infit_MSE_domain",
domain, sep = "")
}
std_outfit_mse_labels <- NULL
for(domain in 1:ndomains){
std_outfit_mse_labels[domain] <- paste("Std.Outfit_MSE_domain",
domain, sep = "")
}
}
names(rater.fit_results) <- c("Rater", outfit_mse_labels, infit_
mse_labels,
std_outfit_mse_labels, std_infit_mse_labels)
rater.fit_results$infit.mean    <-    rowMeans(subset(rater.fit_
results, select = c(Infit_MSE_domain1, Infit_MSE_domain2, Infit_
MSE_domain3, Infit_MSE_domain4)))
rater.fit_results$outfit.mean    <-    rowMeans(subset(rater.fit_
results,
select = c(Outfit_MSE_domain1,
Outfit_MSE_domain2,
Outfit_MSE_domain3,
Outfit_MSE_domain4)))
View(rater.fit_results)
# Request summary statistics
describe(rater.fit_results)
```

In addition to numeric fit statistics, we also constructed scatterplots of standardized residuals associated with individual raters across domains. This analysis corresponds to the approach that we discussed in Chap. 4 for visualizing residuals associated with individual items or persons. We constructed residual scatterplots for the first three raters using the following code. Figure 6.5 includes results for the first three raters; additional raters may be plotted by modifying the raters.to.plot object before the for-loop.

```
raters.to.plot <- c(1:3)
for(rater.number in raters.to.plot){
plot(std.resid.matrix[, rater.number], ylim = c(min.resid,
max.resid),
```

```
main = paste("Standardized Residuals for Rater ",
rater.number, sep = ""),
ylab = "Standardized Residual", xlab = "Domain/Student
Index",
axes = FALSE, xlim = c(1,1460))
box()
grid()
axis(1, labels = NA, tick = FALSE)
axis(2)
abline(h = 0, col = "blue")
abline(h=2, lty = 2, col = "red")
abline(h=-2, lty = 2, col = "red")
abline(v=c(365, 730, 1095))
text(183, 12, "Domain 1")
text(548, 12, "Domain 2")
text(913, 12, "Domain 3")
text(1278, 12, "Domain 4")
legend("bottomright", c("Std. Residual", "Observed =
Expected", "+/- 2 SD"), pch = c(1, NA, NA),
lty = c(NA, 1, 2),
col = c("black", "blue", "red"), cex = .8)
}
```

Table 6.2 includes overall summary statistics for the element-level *MSE* fit statistics for each facet in our MFRM-RS (students, raters, and domains). On average, the fit statistics were within the range of acceptable values for all facets. Table 6.3 includes rater-specific infit *MSE* and outfit *MSE* statistics for the raters in our illustrative data. With the model specification that we used in the TAM R package, *MSE* fit statistics were calculated for each rater specific to each level of the explanatory facet, which in this case is domains. These statistics summarize the residuals associated with each rater's ratings specific to each domain. To facilitate an overall evaluation of the individual raters, we have included an average of the fit statistics associated with each rater along with the domain-specific fit statistics.

Evidence of adequate model-data fit for all facets is essential for the interpretation and use of MFRM parameter estimates as adjusted values that control for differences in rater severity. In practical applications of the MFRM to rater-mediated assessments, it is not always recognized that deviations from acceptable fit for individual raters can compromise the interpretability of student achievement estimates as adjusted for differences in rater severity. In Wind, Engelhard, and Wesolowski (2016), we demonstrated how differences in rater fit to an explanatory Rasch model can prevent meaningful adjustments for rater severity. Figure 6.4 is adapted from Wind et al. (2016) and demonstrates this idea using rater response functions (RRFs), which are rater-analogues to item response functions (IRFs) used with standard Rasch and item response theory models. When raters exhibit good fit to a Rasch model, including the MFRM, a practical consequence is that their RRFs have an invariant ordering such that they do not intersect. As a result, a constant adjustment can be applied to all student achievement parameters to control for differences in rater severity. In

Table 6.2 Summary of parameter estimates and fit from descriptive MFRM-RS

Statistics		Facets		
		Student	Raters	Domains
Location	*M*	0.25	–0.56	0.00
	SD	2.84	0.34	0.67
Standard Error	*M*	0.23	0.05	0.02
	SD	0.07	0.00	0.01
Infit *MSE*	*M*	0.97	0.98	0.98
	SD	1.12	0.17	0.19
Outfit *MSE*	*M*	0.97	0.98	0.98
	SD	0.11	0.18	0.21
Reliability of Separation		0.99	0.98	> 0.99

Fig. 6.4, Rater A and Rater B exhibited different levels of severity, where Rater A was notably more lenient than Rater B. Although these raters differed in severity, they both exhibited good fit to the model. As a result, they had an invariant ordering such that their differences were consistent for all levels of student achievement, and it is possible to apply a constant adjustment to student achievement parameters that controls for these differences.

On the other hand, a practical consequence of rater misfit is that their level of discrimination (i.e., slope) deviates from the model-expected constant value of 1.00. As a result, RRFs may not have an invariant order for all levels of student achievement, and it is not possible to apply a constant adjustment to student achievement parameters that takes into account differences in severity. Figure 6.4 illustrates the practical consequences of rater misfit using Rater C. Like Rater B, Rater C was a relatively severe rater. Rater C also exhibited misfit, which resulted in their slope parameter estimate deviating from the Rasch-expected value. As a result, the relative distance between RRFs for Rater C and good-fitting raters such as Rater A is not consistent across levels of the latent variable.

Specific Rater Errors and Biases

The final special consideration for rater-mediated assessments is rater errors and biases. In addition to general model-data fit considerations, meaningful interpretations and use of rater-mediated assessments requires evidence that rater judgments are not unduly affected by errors and systematic biases. Sometimes referred to as "rater effects" (e.g., Myford & Wolfe, 2003), rater errors and systematic biases are specific patterns of rater judgments that result in examinees receiving a score that is different from the score that is warranted by the quality of their performance. These rating patterns sometimes coincide with rater misfit (see our discussion earlier in

Table 6.3 Summary of rater location estimates and fit from descriptive MFRM-RS

Rater	Location	*SE*	Mean infit *MSE*	Mean outfit *MSE*	Domain-specific infit *MSE*				Domain-specific outfit *MSE*			
					C	O	SF	St	C	O	SF	St
1	–0.19	0.04	0.59	0.55	0.53	0.57	0.63	0.63	0.50	0.54	0.57	0.60
2	–0.02	0.04	1.06	1.05	0.91	1.23	0.90	1.18	0.90	1.25	0.88	1.18
3	–0.01	0.04	0.83	0.82	0.69	1.00	0.77	0.85	0.72	0.97	0.78	0.82
4	0.10	0.04	0.88	0.90	0.72	0.90	0.93	0.96	0.78	0.92	0.95	0.95
5	–0.26	0.04	1.02	1.02	0.99	1.09	1.09	0.90	0.98	1.06	1.14	0.89
6	–0.44	0.04	1.03	1.01	1.05	0.91	1.11	1.05	1.04	0.93	1.02	1.06
7	–0.49	0.04	1.01	1.11	1.05	0.90	0.93	1.18	1.26	0.88	1.01	1.30
8	0.27	0.04	0.98	1.02	0.82	1.12	1.00	1.00	0.88	1.21	0.98	1.03
9	0.75	0.04	0.83	0.82	0.80	0.79	0.80	0.91	0.81	0.76	0.76	0.93
10	–0.48	0.04	1.12	1.20	1.10	1.08	1.03	1.28	1.17	1.11	1.09	1.43
11	–0.08	0.04	1.25	1.23	1.26	1.25	1.32	1.18	1.22	1.18	1.30	1.21
12	–0.17	0.04	0.82	0.80	0.65	0.80	0.95	0.86	0.64	0.77	0.88	0.89
13	0.18	0.04	1.01	1.01	1.06	1.01	0.96	1.01	1.07	0.98	0.89	1.09
14	0.17	0.04	1.27	1.22	1.02	1.31	1.23	1.52	1.00	1.24	1.13	1.49
15	–0.55	0.04	0.98	1.02	0.98	1.00	0.97	0.98	0.97	0.97	1.14	0.98
16	0.42	0.04	0.83	0.81	0.72	0.86	0.96	0.77	0.71	0.83	0.91	0.78
17	0.11	0.04	1.19	1.19	1.19	1.08	1.25	1.22	1.21	1.05	1.23	1.25
18	0.51	0.04	0.99	0.98	0.88	0.94	0.97	1.16	0.91	0.92	0.93	1.18
19	0.07	0.04	1.22	1.23	1.21	1.23	1.21	1.23	1.26	1.22	1.12	1.29
20	0.15	0.04	0.94	0.91	0.90	0.82	1.11	0.95	0.87	0.82	1.04	0.91
21	–0.04	0.16	0.78	0.75	0.72	0.70	0.71	0.98	0.72	0.67	0.68	0.93
M	0.00	0.04	0.98	0.98	0.92	0.98	0.99	1.04	0.93	0.97	0.97	1.06
SD	0.34	0.03	0.17	0.18	0.20	0.19	0.18	0.20	0.21	0.20	0.18	0.22

Note The domains are abbreviated as follows: C = Conventions; O = Organization; SF = Sentence Formation; St = Style

this chapter), but they may also include specific patterns that may not be detected or understood using fit analysis alone.

Researchers have discussed numerous concerns, classification schemes, indicators, and techniques for minimizing the impact of various rater errors and biases. In this section, we provide a brief discussion of several rater errors and systematic biases that are commonly reported and discussed in research using explanatory Rasch models: (1) severity/leniency; (2) range restrictions; and (3) differential rater functioning (DRF), which is related to rater bias. For a detailed discussion of rater errors and systematic biases within the context of explanatory Rasch models, we refer readers to other sources, such as Engelhard and Wind (2018).

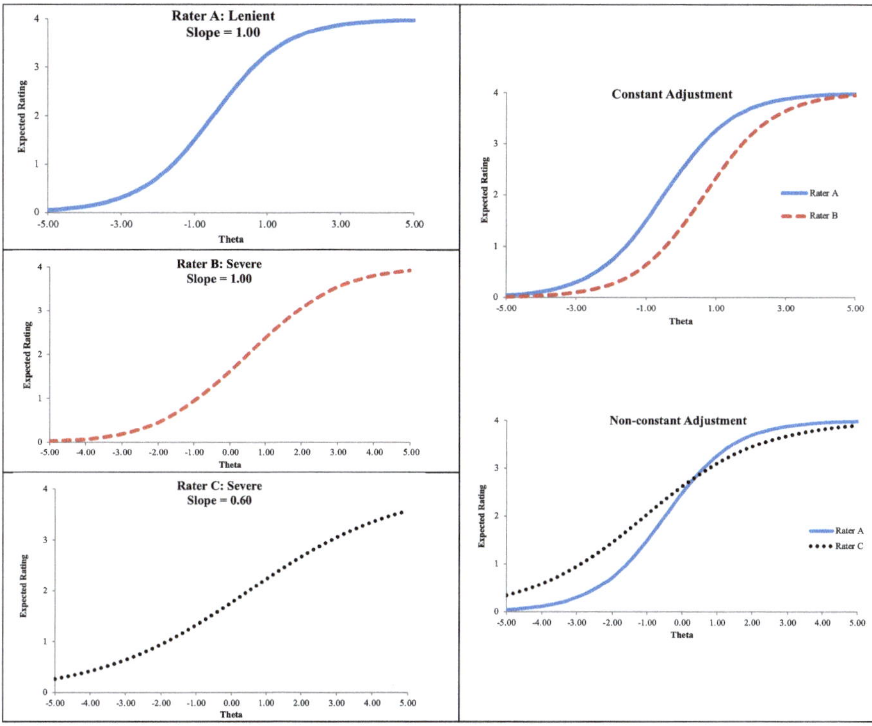

Fig. 6.4 Examples of constant and non-constant adjustments for rater severity

Severity/Leniency

When raters exhibit severity or leniency effects, their ratings are systematically lower or higher than the ratings that are warranted given examinee achievement and task difficulty. Left uncorrected, rater severity and leniency effects can have a clear practical impact on student achievement, especially when they occur in combination with incomplete rating designs. However, assuming adequate model-data fit for raters and sufficient connectivity, the examinee achievement estimates from the MFRM are adjusted to account for rater severity differences. If needed, location parameters for examinees can be transformed back to the original rating scale as an adjusted raw score estimate of achievement. This statistic is sometimes called the "fair average." Reporting the fair average is often useful in practical settings where final examinee scores need to be reported on the original rating scale.

Although adjustments for differences in rater severity are possible and relatively straightforward, it is nevertheless important to identify individual raters within a rater pool who exhibit systematic severity or leniency effects. This information can help researchers understand individual differences among raters to gain a clearer sense of their understanding of the construct and scoring materials. In addition, identifying systematically severe or lenient raters can provide guidance for rater

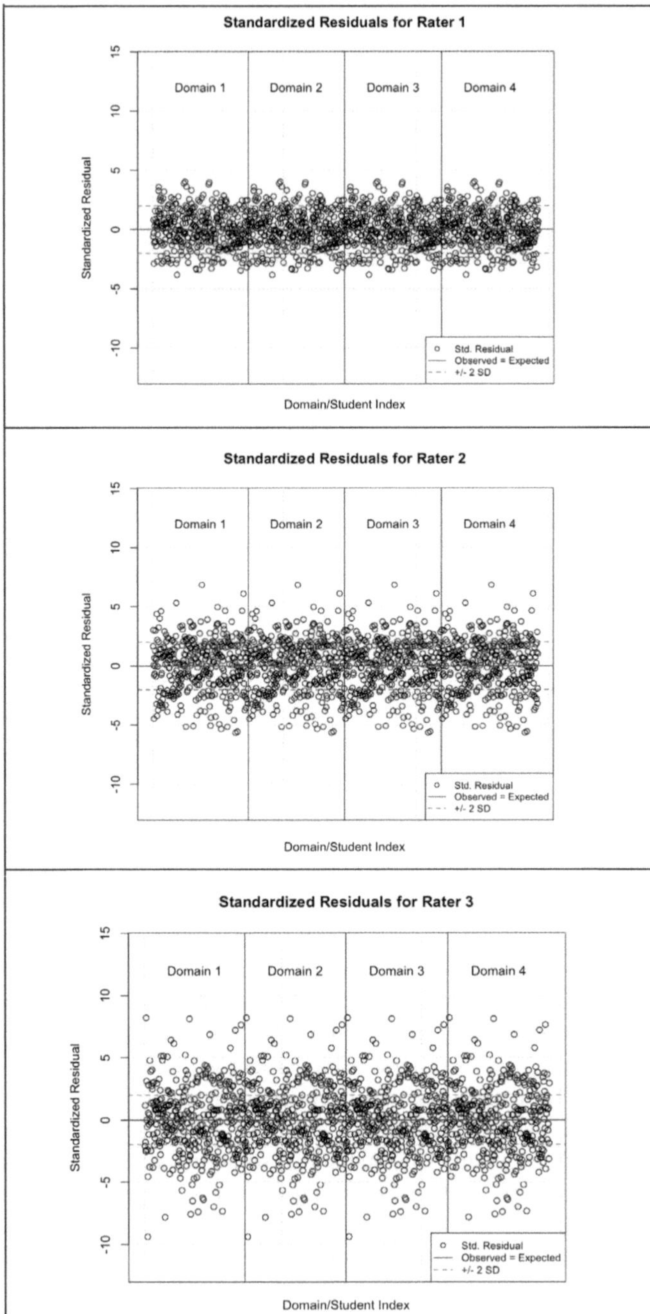

Fig. 6.5 Scatterplots of standardized residuals for individual raters across domains

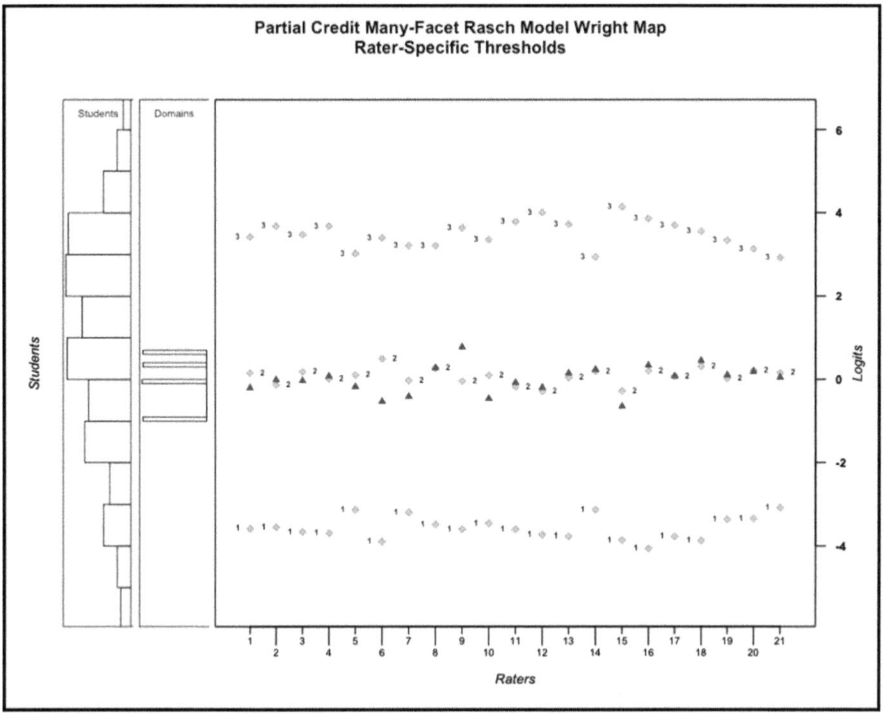

Fig. 6.6 Rater-mediated wright map with rater-specific threshold parameters

training or remediation to help raters develop a more-consistent application of the scoring rubric.

Assuming that rater location estimates are scaled such that the mean is set to zero logits, some researchers have recommended using a critical value of $\lambda > 0.5$ logits to identify raters who exhibit notable severity effects, and $\lambda < -0.5$ logits to identify raters who exhibit notable leniency effects (Myford & Wolfe, 2004; Wolfe & McVay, 2012). Using these criteria to identify severity and leniency effects, three raters would be flagged in our illustrative writing assessment data (see Table 6.3). Specifically, two raters had location parameter estimates higher than 0.5 logits: Rater 9: $\lambda = 0.75$ (*SE* = 0.04) and Rater 18: $\lambda = 0.51$ (*SE* = 0.04), and one rater had a location parameter estimate lower than -0.5 logits: Rater 15: $\lambda = -0.55$ (*SE* = 0.04). Although guidelines such as the 0.5 logit criterion are helpful, context-specific information, such as the use and stakes associated with assessment outcomes, is important when establishing a threshold with which to classify raters as "lenient" or "severe." For example, when training or qualifying raters to score a high-stakes assessment program in which consistent ratings are especially important, researchers may set a lower critical value for identifying rater severity or leniency (e.g., 0.3 logits).

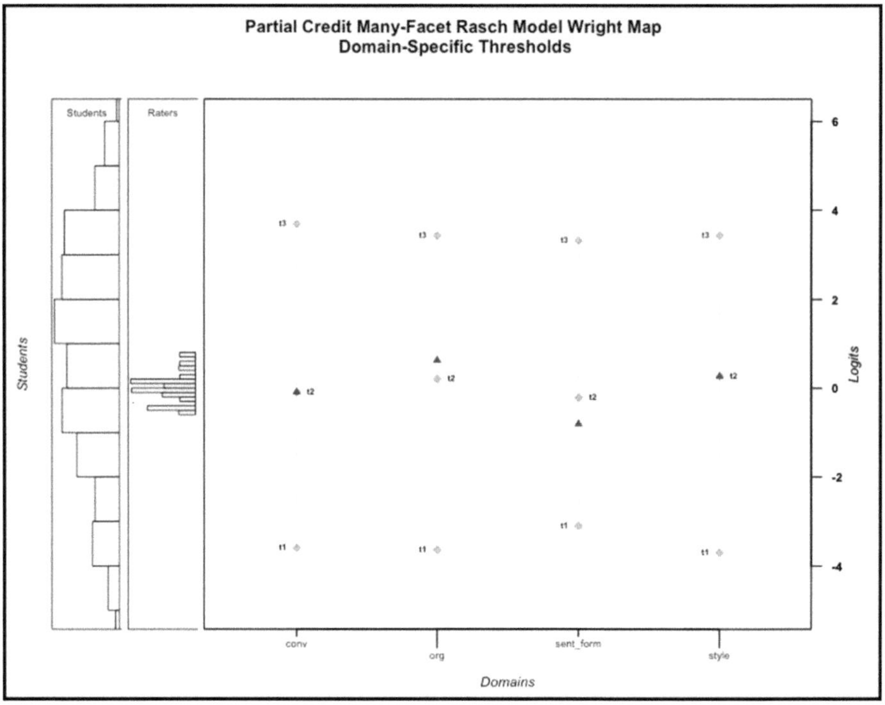

Fig. 6.7 Rater-mediated wright map with domain-specific threshold parameters

Range Restrictions

Next, range restrictions refer to raters' tendencies to assign ratings in a smaller set of rating scale categories than are warranted by the range of examinee achievement. Researchers have discussed and documented several forms of range restrictions, including a tendency to score examinees using only the central category or categories of a rating scale ("centrality" or "central tendency"), and a tendency to score using only the extreme categories in a scale ("extremism"). Researchers have proposed several methods for classifying and identifying range restrictions with the MFRM. Among these methods, some of the most common include model-data fit statistics and analyses of rater-specific threshold estimates calculated using various formulations of the MFRM-PC.

In addition to their general use for evaluating rater fit, infit and outfit *MSE* statistics for individual raters are also sensitive to range restriction effects for individual raters. Relative to the fit statistics for raters who do not exhibit range restrictions, raters who exhibit range restriction effects tend to have low infit and outfit *MSE* statistics. Researchers have noted that infit and outfit are quite sensitive to range restriction effects under a variety of conditions, including incomplete rating designs (Wind & Jones, 2018). However, researchers have also noted that although these fit statistics

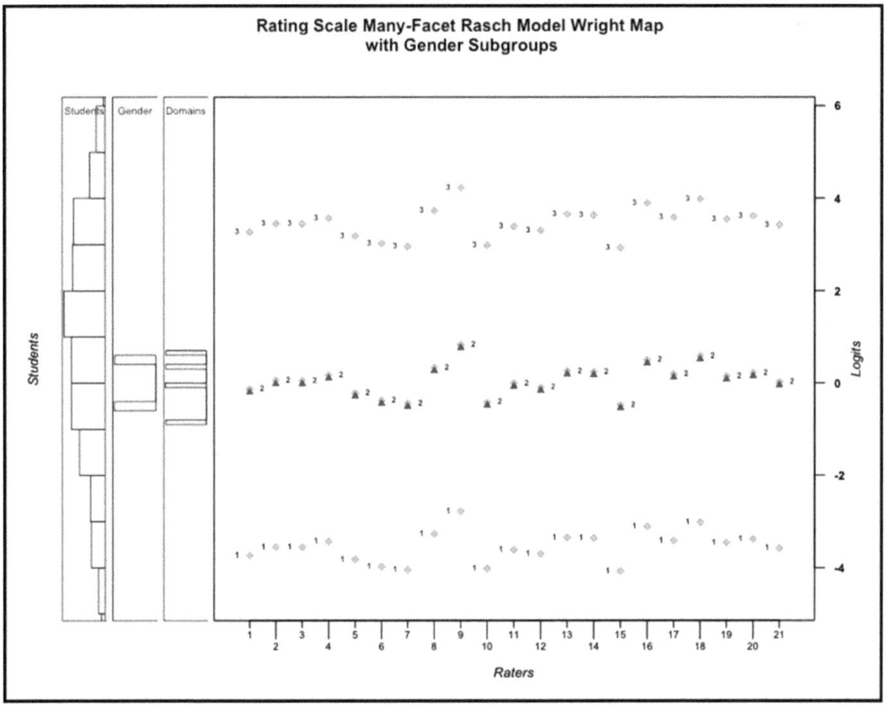

Fig. 6.8 Rater-mediated wright map for a person-explanatory PC-MFRM

are often sensitive to range restrictions such as centrality, they are not specific—that is, raters may have low *MSE* fit statistics for a variety of reasons that include but are not limited to range restrictions (Wolfe & Song, 2015).

A more-direct approach to identifying raters who exhibit range restrictions based on the MFRM is to examine raters' category use directly using statistics specifically related to category use, including the frequency of observations within categories specific to individual raters and the standard deviation (*SD*) of rater-specific threshold parameter estimates.

Table 6.4 provides an overview of rater category use for the Georgia writing assessment data. For each rater, the proportion of ratings observed in each category is presented, along with the proportion of ratings in the central categories ($X = 2$ or $X = 3$) and the extreme categories ($X = 1$ or $X = 4$), and the rater-specific threshold *SD*. On average, the raters tended to use the central categories more often ($M = 0.68$) than the extreme categories ($M = 0.32$). Among the raters in our illustrative data, Rater 12 used the central categories most often (*proportion* = 0.73), and Rater 21 used the extreme categories most often (*proportion* = 0.39). We calculated these proportions and saved them in a matrix for further analysis.

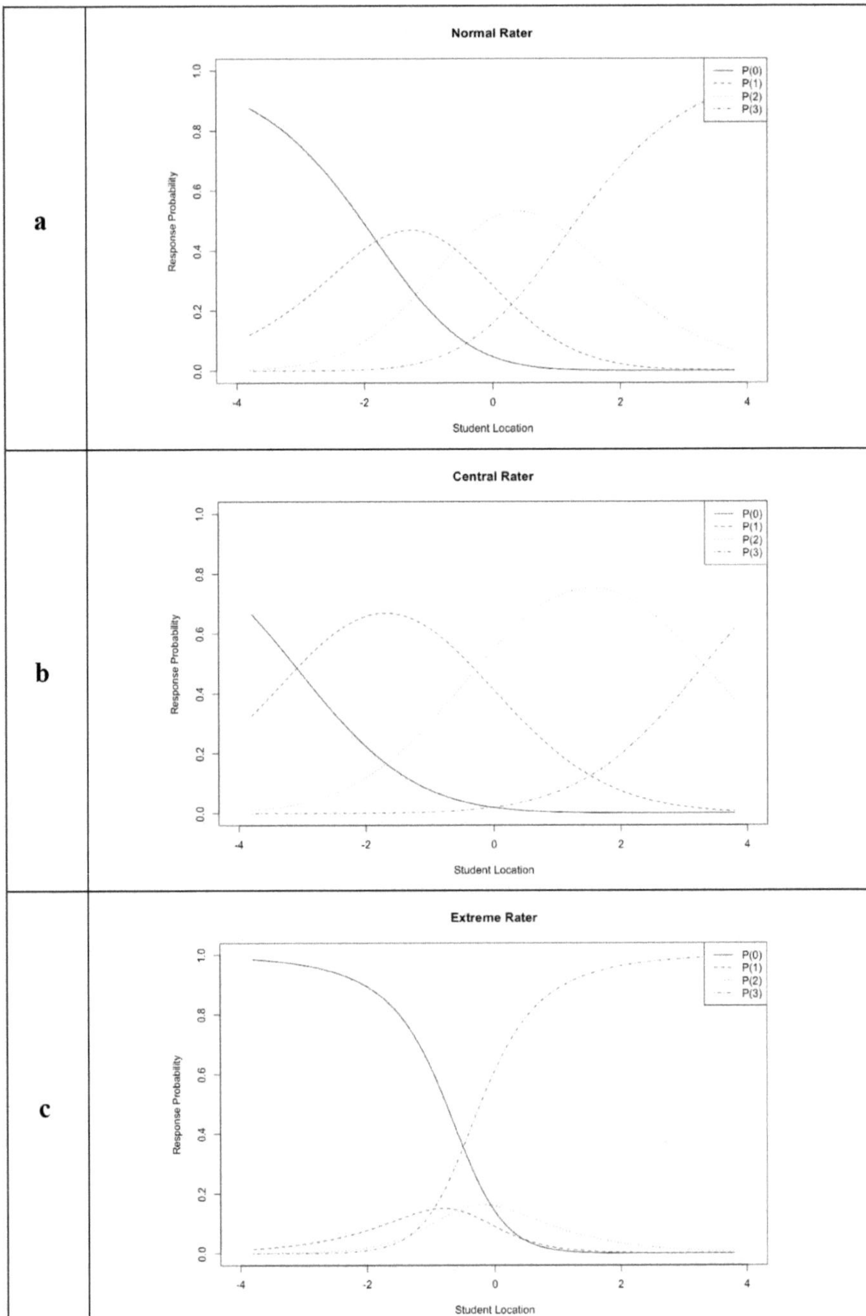

Fig. 6.9 Illustrative category probability curves for a normal rater, central rater, and extreme rater

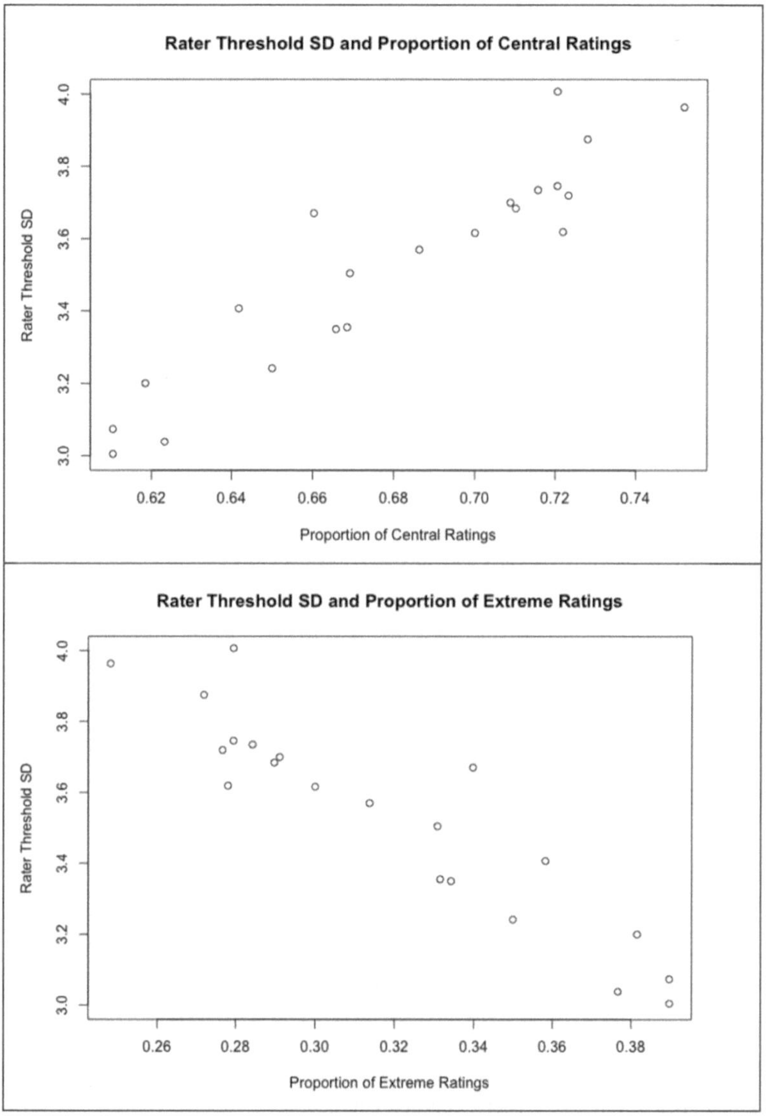

Fig. 6.10 Bivariate relationship between rater threshold SD and raters' use of central and extreme categories

```
## Proportion of ratings in each category:
rater.cat.props <- matrix(data = NA,
nrow = 21,
ncol = 4)
```

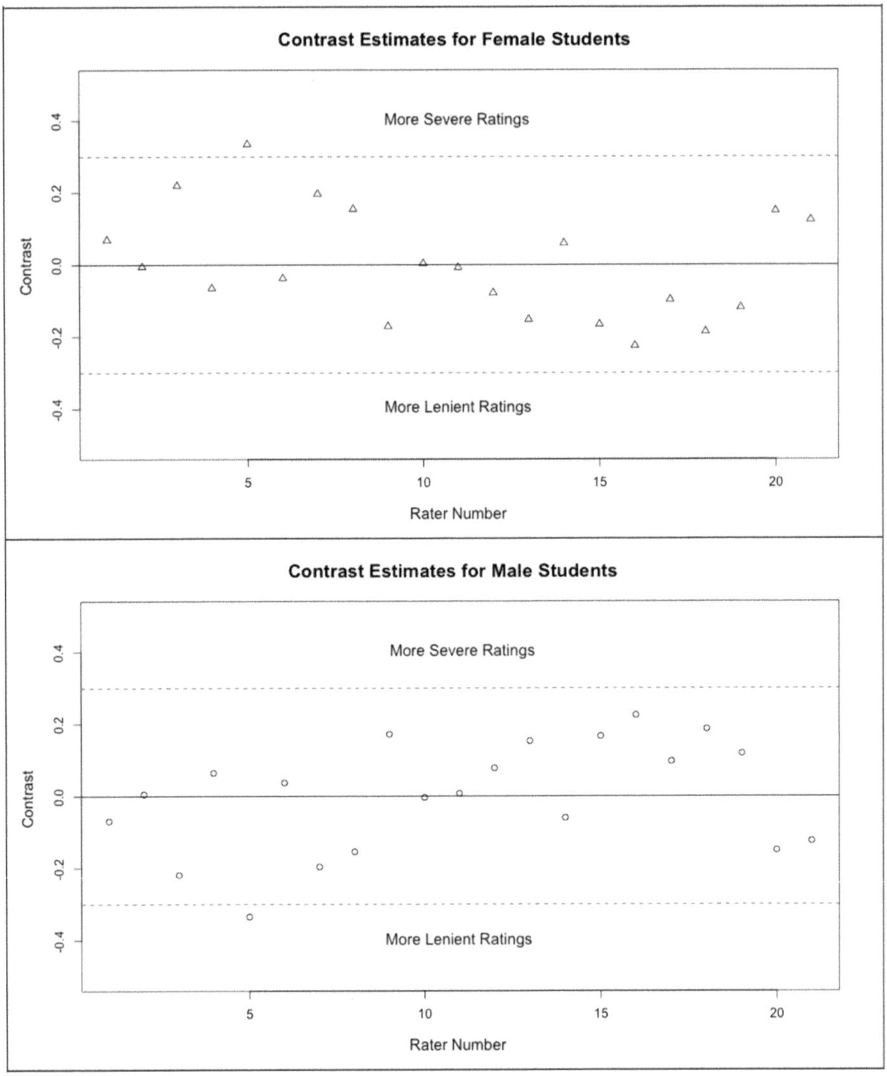

Fig. 6.11 Contrast estimates for rater*subgroup interaction

```
rater.scores <- writing.all[, -c(1:3)]
for(rater.n in 1:21){
rater.cat.props[rater.n,    ]    <-    table(rater.scores[,
rater.n])/sum(table(rater.scores[, rater.n]))
}
rater.cat.props.df <- as.data.frame(rater.cat.props)
names(rater.cat.props.df) <- c("p1", "p2", "p3", "p4")
summary(rater.cat.props.df)
```

Table 6.4 Rater category use for Georgia writing data

Rater	Proportion of ratings within categories				Proportion of ratings in central categories ($X = 2 + X = 3$)	Proportion of ratings in extreme categories ($X = 1 + X = 4$)	Rater threshold *SD*
	$X = 1$	$X = 2$	$X = 3$	X = 4			
1	0.09	0.29	0.38	0.24	0.67	0.33	3.51
2	0.10	0.27	0.43	0.20	0.70	0.30	3.62
3	0.10	0.30	0.38	0.22	0.69	0.31	3.57
4	0.10	0.30	0.41	0.19	0.71	0.29	3.68
5	0.11	0.26	0.35	0.28	0.61	0.39	3.07
6	0.07	0.31	0.35	0.27	0.66	0.34	3.67
7	0.10	0.24	0.37	0.28	0.62	0.38	3.20
8	0.12	0.32	0.35	0.21	0.67	0.33	3.36
9	0.14	0.33	0.40	0.13	0.72	0.28	3.62
10	0.09	0.26	0.38	0.27	0.64	0.36	3.41
11	0.10	0.27	0.44	0.20	0.71	0.29	3.70
12	0.08	0.26	0.47	0.19	0.73	0.27	3.88
13	0.10	0.31	0.41	0.18	0.72	0.28	3.75
14	0.14	0.29	0.33	0.24	0.62	0.38	3.04
15	0.06	0.24	0.48	0.22	0.72	0.28	4.01
16	0.10	0.35	0.40	0.15	0.75	0.25	3.96
17	0.10	0.31	0.41	0.19	0.72	0.28	3.73
18	0.11	0.36	0.37	0.16	0.72	0.28	3.72
19	0.12	0.28	0.38	0.22	0.67	0.33	3.35
20	0.12	0.30	0.35	0.23	0.65	0.35	3.24
21	0.13	0.28	0.33	0.26	0.61	0.39	3.01
Mean	0.10	0.29	0.39	0.21	0.68	0.32	3.53
SD	0.02	0.03	0.04	0.04	0.04	0.04	0.30

Note Ratings were assigned using a scale between 0 and 3, where $X = 0$ indicates "inadequate", $X = 1$ indicates "poor", $X = 2$ indicates "good", and X = 3 indicates "very good".

Next, we calculated rater-specific threshold *SD* values as an indicator of potential range restrictions. To illustrate the logic of the threshold *SD* approach, Fig. 6.9 shows category probability curves for three raters for an assessment with a five-category rating scale: (A) a "normal" rater who does not exhibit range restrictions; (B) a rater who exhibits central tendency by restricting most of their ratings the central categories of the rating scale, and (C) a rater who exhibits extremism by restricting most of their ratings to the extreme categories. When raters limit their responses to central scale categories, the relative distances between their adjacent-categories threshold estimates tend to be wider overall compared to raters who do not limit their responses. Conversely, raters who limit their responses to extreme categories may have very small variability in their threshold locations. Accordingly, researchers can examine the relative distribution of $SD_{\tau r}$ values to identify raters who may exhibit range restrictions.

Returning to our example MFRM specifications earlier in this chapter, Equation 6.3 includes rater-specific thresholds that facilitate analyses related to rater category use. As discussed earlier, we estimated this model in TAM using the wide-format version of the writing assessment data. From the model results, we focused on the rater-specific thresholds as evidence related to raters' category use and potential range restrictions. We calculated rater-specific $SD_{\tau r}$ and examined summary statistics for the results using the matrix of rater-specific thresholds that we generated from the model output as follows.

```
## Threshold SD for individual raters:
rater.threshold.sd <- apply(rater_thresholds, 1, sd)
summary(rater.threshold.sd)
```

To facilitate interpretation of the threshold *SD* values with respect to category use, we plotted the bivariate relationship between rater threshold *SD* and raters' use of the central and extreme categories as reflected in proportions of ratings within categories.

```
## Examine relationship between threshold SD and category use:
rater.cat.props.df$sum.central <- rater.cat.props.df$p2 +
rater.cat.props.df$p3
rater.cat.props.df$sum.extreme <- rater.cat.props.df$p1 +
rater.cat.props.df$p4
rater.cat.props.df$rater.threshold.sd <- rater.threshold.sd
graphics.off()
plot(rater.cat.props.df$sum.central,
rater.cat.props.df$rater.threshold.sd,
ylim = c(3,4), main = "Rater Threshold SD and Proportion of
Central Ratings",
ylab = "Rater Threshold SD", xlab = "Proportion of Central
Ratings")
grid()
plot(rater.cat.props.df$sum.extreme,
rater.cat.props.df$rater.threshold.sd,
ylim = c(3,4), main = "Rater Threshold SD and Proportion of
Extreme Ratings",
ylab = "Rater Threshold SD", xlab = "Proportion of Extreme
Ratings")
grid()
```

Figure 6.10 illustrates the bivariate relationship between rater-specific thresholds and the proportion of ratings in the central and extreme categories. Raters with relatively high values of $SD_{\tau r}$ tended to use the central categories more often (i.e., potential central tendency effects), whereas those with relatively low values of $SD_{\tau r}$ tended to use the extreme categories more often (i.e., potential extremism effects).

Differential Rater Functioning

Finally, differential Rater Functioning (DRF; i.e., rater bias) occurs when raters apply systematically lower or higher levels of severity when they score examinees from different construct-irrelevant subgroups. For example, raters may exhibit DRF related to student gender or linguistic background (e.g., Gyagenda & Engelhard, 2009; Kondo-Brown, 2002; Schaefer, 2008; Winke et al., 2012). Compared to rater severity/leniency effects and range restrictions, DRF is not easily corrected using statistical adjustments and often reflects a notable threat to the fairness of a rater-mediated assessment. Accordingly, it is important that researchers include checks for DRF throughout the assessment process, including during rater training and qualification procedures and operational scoring.

Explanatory Rasch models offer a useful framework in which to identify and explore DRF using interaction effects. For example, the person-explanatory MFRM-RS in Equation 6.7 includes an interaction between rater severity and student subgroup classifications ($\lambda_r\gamma_g$); Fig. 6.8 shows the Wright map that corresponds to this analysis. This type of interaction effect can help researchers identify individual raters who may exhibit DRF related to student subgroups. To illustrate this approach, we applied Equation 6.7 to the example writing assessment data using student gender subgroups. In this model, the interaction term provides an estimate of the degree to which rater severity specific to a student gender subgroup is different from the rater's overall level of severity, after controlling for the latent variable.

We applied the model using the wide-format version of the writing assessment data using the same general procedure as for the previous analyses in this chapter. The following code demonstrates how we prepared the data and specified the model components, which included students, raters, domains, and gender subgroups.

```
## Import the writing assessment data:
writing.all <- read.csv("GA_writing_wide_format.csv")
## Set up the model components:
## Identify the response matrix
#* Note: raters are columns; labeled as "items" by default in
TAM)
ratings <- subset(writing.all, select = c(rater_1 : rater_
21))
ratings.df <- as.data.frame(ratings)
names(ratings.df) <- c(1:21)
## Rescale the ratings to start at zero:
ratings.df.zero <- ratings.df-1
## Specify the facets (domains) in a data frame:
```

```
#* Note: These are facets besides the one
#* represented in columns of the response matrixfacets <-
writing.all[ , c("gender", "domain"), drop = FALSE]
names(facets) <- c("subgroup", "domain")
## Identify the examinee indicators (student ids)
students <- writing.all$student.id
```

We specified the model equation to facilitate the DRF analysis by including an interaction between raters and student subgroups and then estimated the model using the tam.mml.mfr() function.

```
## specify the MFRM in an object ("item" refers to raters)
DRF_equation <- ~ item + subgroup + domain + item*subgroup +
step
DRF_model <- tam.mml.mfr(resp = ratings.df.zero, facets =
facets, formulaA = DRF_equation, pid = students, verbose =
FALSE, constraint = "items")
```

From our DRF model analysis, we focused on rater contrast statistics, which are estimates of the difference between subgroup-specific rater severity estimates and the overall rater severity estimate. Researchers have proposed several critical values for classifying raters based on contrast statistics that reflect different perspectives and assessment contexts. For example, several researchers (e.g., Wind & Guo, 2019; Wolfe & McVay, 2012), have used a value of 0.5 logits for the contrast statistic to identify raters with potentially meaningful DRF. Other researchers have used lower critical values, such as 0.3 logits (e.g., Engelhard & Myford, 2003).

We extracted rater contrast values from the model results and created visual displays to summarize them using the following code.

```
facet.estimates <- DRF_model$xsi.facets
rater.subgroup.interactions <- subset(facet.estimates,
facet.estimates$facet == "item:subgroup")
rater.subgroup.interactions$z <- rater.subgroup.interactions
$xsi/rater.subgroup.interactions$se.xsi
rater.subgroup.interactions$abs.contrast <-
abs(rater.subgroup.interactions$xsi)
## Plot contrast results:
plot(rater.subgroup.interactions$xsi[1:21], ylim = c(-0.5,
0.5),
ylab = "Contrast", xlab = "Rater Number", main = "Contrast
Estimates for Male Students")
abline(h=0)
abline(h=.3, lty = 2, col = "purple")
abline(h=-.3, lty = 2, col = "purple")
grid()
```

```
text(11, .4, "More Severe Ratings")
text(11, -.4, "More Lenient Ratings")
plot(rater.subgroup.interactions$xsi[22:42], ylim = c(-0.5,
0.5),
ylab = "Contrast", xlab = "Rater Number", main = "Contrast
Estimates for Female Students",
pch = 2)
abline(h=0)
abline(h=.3, lty = 2, col = "purple")
abline(h=-.3, lty = 2, col = "purple")
grid()
text(11, .4, "More Severe Ratings")
text(11, -.4, "More Lenient Ratings")
```

Table 6.5 includes contrast estimates for each of the raters in our illustrative dataset specific to the female and male student subgroups; Fig. 6.11 shows these values in separate plots for each subgroup. Because the gender variable in our dataset included two levels, the contrast estimates for the two groups are symmetric. We focused on the magnitude of the contrast estimates to identify raters who exhibited notable differences in severity between subgroups. For all raters, the absolute values of the contrast estimates were below 0.5 in both subgroups. Rater 5 had an absolute contrast statistic of 0.33, with more-severe ratings for male students compared to female students. Overall, the distribution of these contrast statistics suggested small differences between groups, such that the raters tended to exercise a similar level of severity when they scored female and male students' essays.

Discussion and Summary

> Raters are human and they are therefore subject to all of the errors to which humankind must plead guilty (Guilford, 1936, p. 272)

In this chapter, we focused on the use of explanatory Rasch models for rater-mediated assessments. Rater-mediated assessments, unlike selected-response assessments, require human judgment to score constructed responses or performances. We discussed the challenges inherent to rater-mediated assessments, such as subjectivity, potential bias, and the need for consistent rater judgments to ensure reliable, fair and valid measures. We emphasized the concept of rater-invariant measurement that yields ratings of person achievement that is independent of the raters used.

We contrasted traditional methods used to study rater-mediated assessments, such as Generalizability Theory from the Test Score Tradition and Rasch models from the Scaling Tradition. Within the Test Score Tradition, researchers typically focus on evaluating rater reliability or agreement by comparing scores across raters and examinees. The explanatory Rasch model provides a framework to address the unique challenges of rater-mediated assessments, extending invariance principles to rater

Table 6.5 Differential rater functioning results for Georgia writing data

Rater number	Female student contrast	Male student contrast	Absolute value	*SE*	*Z*
1	0.07	–0.07	0.07	0.04	–1.89
2	–0.01	0.01	0.01	0.04	0.14
3	0.22	–0.22	0.22	0.04	–5.99
4	–0.06	0.06	0.06	0.04	1.76
5	0.33	–0.33	0.33	0.04	–9.11
6	–0.04	0.04	0.04	0.04	1.01
7	0.20	–0.20	0.20	0.04	–5.34
8	0.15	–0.15	0.15	0.04	–4.21
9	–0.17	0.17	0.17	0.04	4.70
10	0.00	0.00	0.00	0.04	–0.10
11	–0.01	0.01	0.01	0.04	0.20
12	–0.08	0.08	0.08	0.04	2.12
13	–0.15	0.15	0.15	0.04	4.19
14	0.06	–0.06	0.06	0.04	–1.64
15	–0.17	0.17	0.17	0.04	4.53
16	–0.23	0.23	0.23	0.04	6.19
17	–0.10	0.10	0.10	0.04	2.65
18	–0.19	0.19	0.19	0.04	5.12
19	–0.12	0.12	0.12	0.04	3.25
20	0.15	–0.15	0.15	0.04	–4.07
21	0.12	–0.12	0.12	0.16	–0.76

judgment. An explanatory Rasch model approach involves modeling rater judgments within an invariant measurement framework, considering constructs, persons, and items in the context of rater judgments. We highlighted our earlier work on invariant measurement with raters (Engelhard & Wind, 2018), including our guiding principles for rater-invariant measurement. These principles ensure that the measurement of persons, calibration of cues and rating scales, and the location of raters are independent of the specific raters, persons, and other context-specific assessment components.

We emphasized that the Many-Facet Rasch Model (MFRM; 1989) is an explanatory Rasch model. The MFRM is a valuable practical tool for modeling and controlling rater severity in various disciplinary areas. The MFRM extends the standard Rasch model to include explanatory variables, or facets, related to items, persons, or raters, allowing adjustments for differences in rater severity.

Using the MFRM as the main analytic approach, we discussed special considerations for rater-mediated assessments using an illustrative data analysis from a Georgia High School Writing Test. We focused on three special considerations: data collection designs, parameter interpretations, and specific types of rater errors and biases.

Data collection designs for rater-mediated assessments are typically complex and resource-intensive, often requiring incomplete scoring designs due to practical constraints. Ensuring that student achievement estimates are comparable across different raters is crucial. We considered how explanatory Rasch models can be used to achieve this by separating student achievement estimates from rater severity.

Next, we considered parameter interpretations in explanatory Rasch models for raters. Interpreting parameter estimates in this context helps researchers understand the influence of various facets on the measurement process. For example, the MFRM can include interaction terms to explore how rater severity varies across different student subgroups or assessment components. This approach allows researchers to test hypotheses related to invariance and identify specific rater biases.

In summary, this chapter emphasized the importance of invariant measurement in ensuring the validity, reliability, and fairness of rater-mediated assessment systems. By using explanatory Rasch models, researchers can address the unique challenges of rater judgment and improve the overall quality of assessment outcomes.

References

Andrich, D. A. (2018). Rasch rating-scale model. In W. J. van der Linden (Ed.), *Handbook of Item Response Theory* (Vol. 1, pp. 31–50). CRC Press.

Engelhard, G. (1997). Constructing rater and task banks for performance assessments. *Journal of Outcome Measurement, 1*(1), 19–33.

Engelhard, G., & Myford, C. M. (2003). *Monitoring faculty consultant performance in the Advanced Placement English Literature and Composition Program with a many-faceted Rasch model.* College Entrance Examination Board.

Engelhard, G., & Wind, S. A. (2018). *Invariant measurement with raters and rating scales: Rasch models for rater-mediated assessments.* Taylor & Francis.

Guilford, J. P. (1936). *Psychometric methods.* McGraw-Hill.

Gyagenda, I. S., & Engelhard, G. (2009). Using classical and modern measurement theories to explore rater, domain, and gender influences on student writing ability. *Journal of Applied Measurement, 10*(3), 225–246.

Hombo, C. M., Donoghue, J. R., & Thayer, D. T. (2001). *A simulation study of the effect of rater designs on ability estimation* (ETS Research Report RR-01-05). Educational Testing Service.

Johnson, R. L., Penny, J. A., & Gordon, B. (2009). *Assessing performance: Designing, scoring, and validating performance tasks.* The Guilford Press.

Jones, E., & Wind, S. A. (2018). Using repeated rating occasions to improve measurement precision in incomplete rating designs. *Journal of Applied Measurement, 19*(2), 148–161.

Kaliski, P. K., Wind, S. A., Engelhard, G., Morgan, D. L., Plake, B. S., & Reshetar, R. A. (2013). Using the Many-Faceted Rasch Model to evaluate standard setting judgments: An illustration with the advanced placement environmental science exam. *Educational and Psychological Measurement, 73*(3), 386–411. https://doi.org/10.1177/0013164412468448

Kirk, R. E. (1995). *Experimental design: Procedures for the behavioral sciences* (3rd ed.). Brooks/Cole.

Knoch, U., Read, J., & von Randow, J. (2007). Re-training writing raters online: How does it compare with face-to-face training? *Assessing Writing, 12*(1), 26–43. https://doi.org/10.1016/j.asw.2007.04.001

Kondo-Brown, K. (2002). A FACETS analysis of rater bias in measuring Japanese second language writing performance. *Language Testing, 19*(1), 3–31. https://doi.org/10.1191/0265532202lt218oa

Linacre, J. M. (1989). *Many-Facet Rasch Measurement*. MESA Press.

Lumley, T., & McNamara, T. F. (1995). Rater characteristics and rater bias: Implications for training. *Language Testing, 1995*(12), 54–71.

Masters, G. N. (1982). A Rasch model for partial credit scoring. *Psychometrika, 47*(2), 149–174. https://doi.org/10.1007/BF02296272

McNamara, T., & Knoch, U. (2012). The Rasch wars: The emergence of Rasch measurement in language testing. *Language Testing, 29*(4), 555–576. https://doi.org/10.1177/0265532211430367

Myford, C. M., & Wolfe, E. W. (2000). Strengthening the ties that bind: Improving the linking network in sparsely connected rating designs. *ETS Research Report Series, 2000*(1), i–34. https://doi.org/10.1002/j.2333-8504.2000.tb01832.x

Myford, C. M., & Wolfe, E. W. (2003). Detecting and measuring rater effects using many-facet Rasch measurement: Part I. *Journal of Applied Measurement, 4*(4), 386–422.

Myford, C. M., & Wolfe, E. W. (2004). Detecting and measuring rater effects using many-facet Rasch measurement: Part II. *Journal of Applied Measurement, 5*(2), 189–227.

Raczynski, K. R., Cohen, A. S., Engelhard, G., Jr., & Lu, Z. (2015). Comparing the effectiveness of self-paced and collaborative frame-of-reference training on rater accuracy in a large-scale writing assessment. *Journal of Educational Measurement, 52*(3), 301–318.

Revelle, W. (2016). *psych: Procedures for Personality and Psychological Research (1.6.9)*. [Computer software]. Northwestern University. https://CRAN.R-project.org/package=psych

Robitzsch, A., Kiefer, T., & Wu, M. (2020). *TAM: Test Analysis Modules* (3.5-19) [Computer software]. https://CRAN.R-project.org/package=TAM

Saal, F. E., Downey, R. G., & Lahey, M. A. (1980). Rating the ratings: Assessing the psychometric quality of rating data. *Psychological Bulletin 88*(2), 413–428.

Schaefer, E. (2008). Rater bias patterns in an EFL writing assessment. *Language Testing, 25*(4), 465–493. https://doi.org/10.1177/0265532208094273

Schumacker, R. E. (1999). Many-facet Rasch Analysis with crossed, nested, and mixed designs. *Journal of Outcome Measurement, 3*(4), 323–338.

Torres Irribarra, D., & Freund, R. (2014). *Wright Map: IRT item-person map with ConQuest integration* [Computer software]. http://github.com/david-ti/wrightmap

Wesolowski, B. C., & Wind, S. A. (2019). Pedagogical considerations for examining rater variability in rater-mediated assessments: A three-model framework. *Journal of Educational Measurement, 56*(3), 521–546.

Williamson, D. M., Xi, X., & Breyer, F. J. (2012). A Framework for Evaluation and Use of Automated Scoring. *Educational Measurement: Issues and Practice, 31*(1), 2–13. https://doi.org/10.1111/j.1745-3992.2011.00223.x

Wind, S. A., Engelhard, G., & Wesolowski, B. (2016). Exploring the effects of rater linking designs and rater fit on achievement estimates within the context of music performance assessments. *Educational Assessment, 21*(4), 278–299. https://doi.org/10.1080/10627197.2016.1236676

Wind, S. A., & Ge, Y. (2021). Detecting Rater Biases in Sparse Rater-Mediated Assessment Networks. *Educational and Psychological Measurement, 0013164420988108*. https://doi.org/10.1177/0013164420988108

Wind, S. A., & Guo, W. (2019). Exploring the combined effects of rater misfit and differential rater functioning in performance assessments. *Educational and Psychological Measurement*, 0013164419834613. https://doi.org/10.1177/0013164419834613

Wind, S. A., & Jones, E. (2017). The Stabilizing Influences of Linking Set Size and Model?Data Fit in Sparse Rater-Mediated Assessment Networks. *Educational and Psychological Measurement, 001316441770373*. https://doi.org/10.1177/0013164417703733

Wind, S. A., & Jones, E. (2018). Exploring the influence of range restrictions on connectivity in sparse assessment networks: An illustration and exploration within the context of classroom observations. *Journal of Educational Measurement, 55*(2), 217–242.

Wind, S. A., & Jones, E. (2019a). Not Just Generalizability: A Case for Multifaceted Latent Trait Models in Teacher Observation Systems. *Educational Researcher, 48*(8), 521–533. https://doi.org/10.3102/0013189X19874084

Wind, S. A., & Jones, E. (2019b). The effects of incomplete rating designs in combination with rater effects. *Journal of Educational Measurement, 56*(1), 76–100. https://doi.org/10.1111/jedm.12201

Winke, P., Gass, S., & Myford, C. (2012). Raters' L2 background as a potential source of bias in rating oral performance. *Language Testing, 30*(2), 231–252. https://doi.org/10.1177/0265532212456968

Wolfe, E. W. (2004). Equating and item banking with the Rasch model. In E. V. Smith & R. M. Smith (Eds.), *Introduction to Rasch measurement*. JAM Press.

Wolfe, E. W., & McVay, A. (2012). Application of Latent Trait Models to Identifying Substantively Interesting Raters. *Educational Measurement: Issues and Practice, 31*(3), 31–37. https://doi.org/10.1111/j.1745-3992.2012.00241.x

Wolfe, E. W., & Song, T. (2015). Comparison of models and indices for detecting rater centrality. *Journal of Applied Measurement, 16*(3), 228–241.

Chapter 7
Instrument Development with Explanatory Rasch Models

Test development requires a systematic approach to ensure the validity of test score interpretations and uses based on those interpretations

(Lane et al., 2015, p. 3).

So far in this book, we have discussed and illustrated various forms of explanatory Rasch models, with an emphasis on components of the model, model evaluation, and interpretation of results from model estimation. In Chap. 7, we discuss and illustrate how explanatory Rasch models can support instrument development for measurement across a variety of contexts. We start with a theoretical discussion of instrument development informed by the measurement, explanation, and invariance principles introduced in Chap. 2. Then, we present an illustrative data analysis with Transitive Reasoning assessment data to demonstrate the use of explanatory Rasch models in this process. We include a second illustration using data from a biology assessment. We end the chapter with a synthesis and discussion of the key ideas.

Five Components for Instrument Development

Figure 7.1 illustrates a process for instrument development that is based on five components that reflect measurement, explanation, and invariance principles. The process includes five interacting components in a cyclical process that are informed by aspects of the measurement context, reflected in the cloud surrounding the five components. The purpose of Fig. 7.1 is to highlight how each component of the instrument development process is influenced by the measurement context, as well as how the components interact with one another to inform next steps. This process incorporates ideas from the constructing measures frameworks proposed and discussed in previous research (Engelhard & Wang, 2021; Wilson, 2005, 2023) with an added emphasis on structural aspects that reflect explanatory Rasch models.

G. Engelhard and S. A. Wind, *Invariant Measurement with Explanatory Rasch Models in the Human Sciences*, https://doi.org/10.1007/978-3-032-08816-1_7

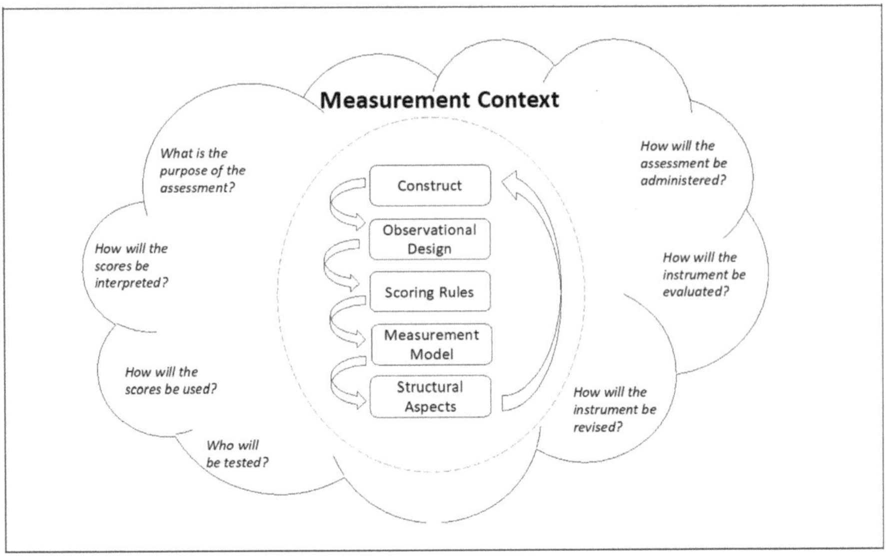

Fig. 7.1 Five components for instrument development

Instrument development cannot be completed within a vacuum. Instead, it requires explicit consideration of contextual factors. These contextual factors are relevant at each stage in the instrument development process. Contextualized instrument development requires researchers to consider and address several practical questions. The large cloud surrounding the 5 components of the instrument development process in Fig. 7.1 includes examples of some of these questions. For example, researchers should consider:

What is the purpose of the assessment?

How will the scores be interpreted?

How will the scores be used?

Who will be tested?

How will the assessment be administered?

How will the instrument be evaluated?

How will the instrument be revised?

Table 7.1 provides guiding questions related to each of the five components for instrument development from Fig. 7.1. For each component, we present an overall guiding question and questions that reflect item-specific and person-specific considerations. In the following sections, we discuss these questions and other ideas related to each of the five components. Reflecting the focus of this book, we devote the most attention to the Measurement Model and Structural Aspects components, while acknowledging that the preceding components and contextual considerations are critical to developing and appropriately using measurement instruments.

Table 7.1 Five components for instrument development

Components	Guiding Questions		
	Overall	Items	Persons
Construct	What is the construct being measured?	What is the expected order of items in terms of more or less of the construct?	What is the expected order of persons in terms of more or less of the construct?
Observational design	What is the plan for collecting structured responses or observations from persons?	What are the item characteristics used to define the construct (e.g., content, cognitive levels)?	What are the key characteristics of the persons in the sample (e.g., age, gender)?
Scoring rules	How are responses or observations categorized to represent item and person locations on the construct?	How are scores assigned to different item types?	Are different scoring rules used for subgroups of persons (e.g., disabilities, language proficiency)?
Measurement model	How are person and item responses or observations mapped onto the construct?	Do the locations of the items match the order expected based on the construct?	Do the locations of the persons match the order expected based on the construct?
Structural aspects	What are the relationships examined?	Do item covariates support our understanding of the construct?	Do the person covariates support our understanding of the construct?

Construct

The first component in our instrument development process is the construct (i.e., latent variable). Instrument development requires researchers to identify and define the construct that the instrument is intended to measure. Visualization tools such as construct maps (Wilson, 2005, 2024) are particularly helpful for defining and delimiting the construct. Construct maps are visual displays that illustrate a construct using a linear continuum. The linear continuum highlights the progression of the construct with respect to person characteristics and item characteristics.

Figure 1.1 from Chapter 1 highlights the progression of a construct along a linear continuum where person locations range from low to high and item locations range from easy to hard. Reflecting the item-related and person-related guiding questions in Table 7.1, the construct map includes item classifications and person characteristics as explanatory variables that provide additional insight into person and item ordering on the underlying continuum that defines the construct. Using guidance from previous literature and theory, along with context-specific considerations, can help researchers identify the expected order of individual items or item characteristics, as well as individual persons or person characteristics on the construct.

Observational Design

The second component in the instrument development process is Observational Design. As shown in Table 7.1, the overall question guiding this component is: What is the plan for collecting structured responses or observations from persons? The Observational Design component involves identifying appropriate procedures with which to systematically observe the construct. For example, researchers may develop multiple-choice items, a scoring rubric, or an observation protocol whose components reflect key aspects from the Construct Map. In terms of item-specific considerations, creating an observational design for an instrument requires researchers to identify the item characteristics that are essential for defining the construct. For example, item characteristics may include content features or cognitive levels that reflect different aspects or levels of the construct. Research related to task modeling and assessment engineering (Embretson, 2023; Luecht, 2013, 2025) is connected to these item-related considerations for the Observational Design component of the instrument development process.

In terms of person-specific considerations, the observational design component involves considering how person-related characteristics should be considered during sampling and data collection. As shown in Table 7.1, researchers should identify the key characteristics of the intended population of test-takers. Such characteristics may reflect demographic variables that are often reported in social science research (e.g., age, gender). Person-related characteristics may also include context-specific variables, such as different levels or frequency of experiences relevant to a particular construct.

Scoring Rules

The third component in the instrument design process is Scoring Rules. This component involves classifying the qualitative observations collected through the observational design (e.g., item responses or rater scores) within ordinal categories that reflect the progression of the construct as a linear continuum. As shown in Table 7.1, the overall guiding question for the scoring rules component is: How are responses or observations categorized to represent item and person locations on the construct?

For example, in an assessment with multiple-choice items, researchers may classify one response option as "correct"—indicating a higher level of achievement and the others as "incorrect"—indicating lower levels of achievement. In a performance assessment, researchers may provide descriptions of score categories that reflect increasing levels of control or understanding of a construct. For an affective scale with selected-response items, researchers may classify certain responses (e.g., "Strongly Disagree") as reflecting lower levels of the construct than other responses (e.g., "Strongly Agree").

With respect to item-specific considerations, defining scoring rules requires researchers to determine how scores are assigned to items with different characteristics. For example, researchers need to consider the degree to which unique scoring rules are needed for items with different characteristics. Items with certain characteristics may need to be scored differently than those with other characteristics. Likewise, researchers also need to consider the degree to which scoring rules hold for all members of the test-taker population. In some cases, scoring rules may need to be adapted for persons with certain characteristics, such as language background or proficiency or disability status.

Measurement Model

The fourth component of the instrument design process is the Measurement Model used to analyze scored responses. The measurement model provides the mechanism through which item and person responses translate to measures on a continuum that reflects the construct. In this book, we focus on measurement models situated within the Rasch measurement theory framework. When model requirements are satisfied, model-derived estimates for items, persons, and associated covariates can be expressed on a single continuum.

After the measurement model is applied, researchers can use the results to consider the alignment between item-related and person-related expectations or hypotheses identified during earlier stages in the instrument development process. As outlined in Table 7.1, researchers can consider the degree to which the empirical order of item locations estimated with the measurement model corresponds to the order that was expected based on the construct map. Similarly, for persons, researchers can compare the observed order of person locations to what was expected based on the construct map. Deviations from these expectations can help researchers identify areas for revision or further investigation with respect to items, persons, or theory related to the construct. We consider various measurement model specifications and interpretations in more detail in our illustrations later in this chapter.

Structural Aspects

The fifth component in the instrument design process is Structural Aspects. This component highlights the role of item- and person-related explanatory variables that have been a major point of emphasis throughout this book. In this component of the instrument design process, researchers identify the relationships associated with specific item- or person-related covariates that should be examined to inform the interpretation, use, and revision of a measurement instrument.

For item-related covariates, researchers can examine location estimates and indicators of measurement quality (e.g., model-data fit) with respect to the expected order on the construct based on the construct map and consider how model results support research and practice related to the construct. Similarly, for persons, researchers can consider how estimates associated with person-related covariates align with hypotheses and expectations, and the degree to which empirical results provide direction to support additional investigation or inform practice.

Illustration One: Transitive Reasoning Assessment

Following the structure of Fig. 7.1 and Table 7.1, this section includes an illustration of the components for instrument development using analyses with Transitive Reasoning assessment data. Table 7.2 provides an overview of the components for instrument development applied to the Transitive Reasoning assessment. Reflecting the focus of our book, we provide a brief discussion of the first three components before focusing on the Measurement Model and Structural Aspects components with detailed illustrations.

Construct

The Transitive Reasoning assessment was designed to measure student ability to reason about relationships (e.g., equality, inequality) between physical objects (e.g., balls, cubes, disks, and sticks) with respect to their physical properties (e.g., length, weight, or area). The assessment instrument included ten items with different characteristics with respect to relationship, type of object, and physical properties. The items reflected transitive reasoning tasks that involved either three or four objects. Table 7.3 provides an overview of the item characteristics and classifications. Broadly speaking, children with higher levels of transitive reasoning are expected to correctly reason about more complex transitive relations more often than children with lower levels of transitive reasoning. According to developmental theories (Bouwmeester & Sijtsma, 2004), children in lower grade levels are generally expected to have lower levels of transitive reasoning compared to those in higher grade levels. Likewise, items involving more objects and more-complex relationships are expected to be harder than those with fewer objects and less-complex relationships.

Figure 7.2 provides an example of a construct map that could be used along with the Transitive Reasoning assessment. The left side of the figure reflects person (student)-related hypotheses, and the right side of the figure reflects task (item)-related hypotheses. Because we are not content-area experts in transitive reasoning, we have not identified an expected progression for individual students or individual tasks; rather, we used smiley-faces to represent our sample of students and puzzle pieces to represent the 10 items in the assessment. The construct map illustrates our hypotheses with respect to the progression of student achievement in transitive reasoning between grade levels, where we expect that students in higher grade levels will demonstrate higher levels of achievement in transitive reasoning. Likewise, we expect that tasks involving fewer objects (3 objects) will be easier to solve correctly compared to those with more objects (4 objects).

Table 7.2 Components for instrument development applied to the transitive reasoning assessment

Components	Questions	Overall	Items	Persons
Construct	What is the construct being measured?	Transitive reasoning	Tasks involving fewer objects are expected to be easier to solve correctly.	Students in higher grade levels are expected to solve tasks more easily.
Observational design	What is the plan for collecting structured responses or observations from persons?	Selected-response items administered to students	Items developed based on developmental theory about transitive reasoning	Person characteristics identified based on theory about transitive reasoning
Scoring rules	How are responses or observations categorized to represent person locations on the latent variable?	Item responses scored for correctness	Items categorized based on number of items	Student subgroups based on grade levels
Measurement model	How are person and item responses or observations mapped onto the latent variable?	Dichotomous Rasch Model	LLRM	LLRM
Structural aspects	What are the relationships examined?	Student achievement and item difficulty	Item covariates estimated and used to examine predicted theoretical implications	Person covariates estimated and used to examine predicted theoretical implications

Observational Design

Each of the ten tasks in the Transitive Reasoning assessment required students to reason about the relationships between some number of objects with respect to a physical property (see Table 7.3). Student responses were scored as either correct or incorrect according to an item-specific rubric.

Table 7.3 Transitive reasoning item classifications

Task number	Physical property (Y)	Format	Objects	Measures	Number of objects
1	Length	$Y_A > Y_B > Y_C$	Sticks	12, 11.5, 11 (cm)	3
2	Length	$Y_A = Y_B = Y_C = Y_D$	Tubes	12 (cm)	4
3	Weight	$Y_A > Y_B > Y_C$	Tubes	45, 25, 27 (g)	3
4	Weight	$Y_A = Y_B = Y_C = Y_D$	Cubes	65 (g)	4
5	Weight	$Y_A < Y_B < Y_C$	Balls	40, 50, 70 (g)	3
6	Area	$Y_A > Y_B > Y_C$	Discs	2.5, 7, 6.5 (diameter; cm)	3
7	Length	$Y_A > Y_B = Y_C$	Sticks	27.5, 27.5, 27.5 (cm)	3
7	Weight	$Y_A > Y_B = Y_C$	Balls	65, 40, 40 (g)	3
9	Length	$Y_A = Y_B < Y_C = Y_D$	Sticks	12.5, 12.5, 13, 13 (cm)	4
10	Weight	$Y_A = Y_B < Y_C = Y_D$	Balls	60, 60, 100, 100 (g)	4

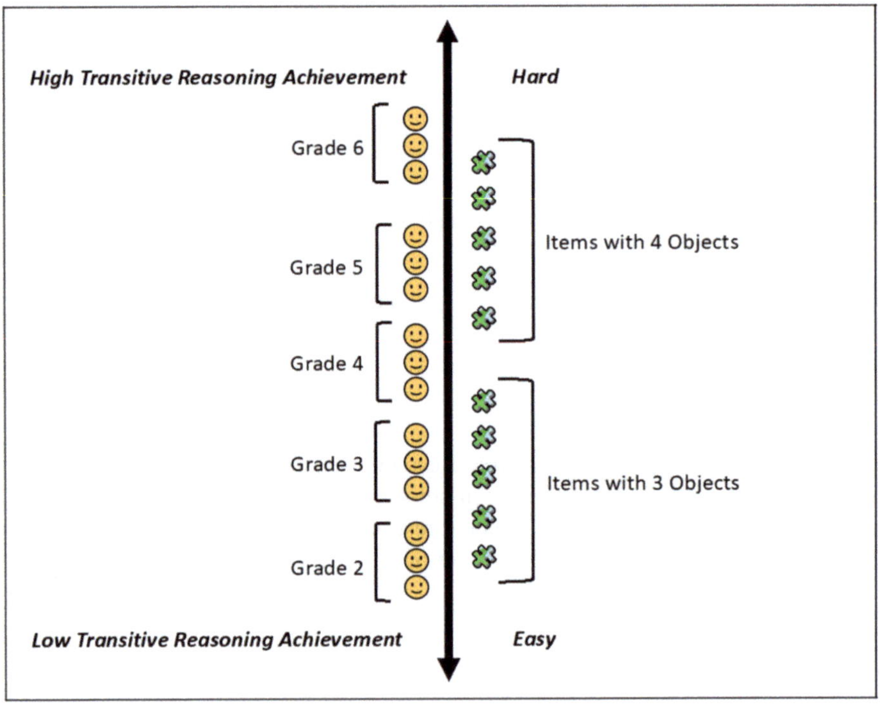

Fig. 7.2 Sample construct map for transitive reasoning assessment

Scoring Rules

Student responses that indicated a correct understanding of the transitive relationships between objects received a score of "1". Those that were incorrect received a score of "0". Students with more-frequent correct scores were interpreted as exhibiting higher levels of transitive reasoning achievement compared to those with less-frequent correct scores.

Measurement Model

The measurement model is the dichotomous Rasch model.

Structural Aspects

Our illustrative analysis uses two models with different specifications that reflect different structural considerations relevant to the Transitive Reasoning Assessment. These two models are (1) the LLRM (also referred to as LLTM), which serves as an item-explanatory model, and (2) the LRRM, which serves as a person-explanatory model. We conducted the analyses using functions from base R, lme4 (Bates et al., 2024), and WrightMap (Torres Irribarra & Freund, 2014). We provide R code examples to illustrate our approach.

Data Preparation for Transitive Reasoning

Several steps were required to prepare the transitive reasoning data for analysis with the dichotomous Rasch model and extended models. First, we loaded the required packages and set the working directory to the location in which we stored the data file. Then, we imported the data.

```
# Prepare for the analysis
## Load required packages:
library(lme4)
library(psych)
library(WrightMap)
## Set the working directory:
setwd("~/Documents/Wind/GE SW Explanatory Models Book/
extended models for raters and ratings/chapter 7")
## Import the transitive reasoning data:
```

```
transreas <-read.csv("transreas.csv")
```

The original transitive reasoning data file is structured in wide format, such that each row includes a single student's identification number, grade level, and responses to tasks 1 through 10. To apply functions from the lme4 package to estimate the base and extended Rasch models using a generalized linear modeling (GLM) approach, it was necessary to re-shape the data from wide to long format, such that multiple rows appear for each student with their response to each item. We used the reshape () function from base R. After re-shaping the data, we sorted it by student and item indicator to facilitate further analyses.

```
## Reshape the data to long format:
transreas_long <- reshape(data = transreas,
direction = "long",
varying = 3:12,
timevar = "item",
v.names = "response",
idvar = "student")
## Re-order the data by Student id and item indicator
transreas_long.ordered <- transreas_long[order(transreas_
long$student,
transreas_long$item),]
```

In preparation for our analyses with item covariates, we added a variable to the sorted data in which we identified the number of items associated with each transitive reasoning task. We stored these item characteristics in a factor variable called n.objects.

```
## Add item classifications
n.objects <- c(3, 4, 3, 4, 3, 3, 3, 3, 4, 4)
transreas_long.ordered$n.objects <- as.factor(n.objects)
```

As a final step in preparing the data for analysis using functions from lme4, we converted the item indicator and student grade level indicator variables to factors.

```
# Convert the item indicator variable to a factor
transreas_long.ordered$item.f    <-    as.factor(transreas_
long.ordered$item)
# Convert the grade level indicator variable to a factor:
transreas_long.ordered$grade.f    <-    as.factor(transreas_
long.ordered$Grade)
```

Model 1: Dichotomous Rasch Model

Reflecting the dichotomous item scores in the transitive reasoning assessment, the base model for our analysis is the dichotomous Rasch model. Using the language of GLMs and explanatory Rasch models, the dichotomous Rasch model can be viewed as a descriptive model with random effects for persons (in this case, students), and fixed effects for items.

We specified the settings for analysis with the lme4 functions and then estimated the dichotomous Rasch model using the glmer() function with the appropriate settings.

```
######## 1. Base model: Random Students, Fixed Items ########
# Adjust settings for analyses:
control=glmerControl(optimizer = "optimx", calc.derivs =
FALSE,
optCtrl = list(method = "nlminb", starttests = FALSE, kkt =
FALSE))
```

We estimated the model using the glmer function. We specified students as a random effect using the syntax (1|Student). We stored results from the analysis in a model object labeled m1.

```
# Estimate the model:
m1 <- glmer(response ~ -1 + item.f + (1|Student),
family = binomial("logit"),
data = transreas_long.ordered,
control = control)
```

Next, we extracted item parameters from the model results. With the glmer function from lme4, item locations are calculated as item easiness. For a more familiar interpretation, we multiplied the values by -1 to convert them to item difficulty.

```
# Extract fixed item parameters:
m1.fixed_items <- data.frame(easiness = fixef(m1))
## Sort the items by location:
m1.fixed_items$item.n <- 1:10
m1.fixed_items.ordered <- m1.fixed_items[order(-m1.fixed_
items$easiness),]
## Convert item easiness to item difficulty:
m1.fixed_items.ordered$difficulty <- m1.fixed_
items.ordered$easiness*-1
```

To understand the distribution of item locations, we calculated summary statistics on the item difficulty parameters. We used the describe() function from the psych package to generate these statistics.

```
## Calculate summary statistics for item difficulty:
summary(m1.fixed_items.ordered$difficulty)
```

The average item difficulty location was equal to -1.93 logits ($SD = 1.56$), with a range from -4.05 to 5.06 logits. To visualize these results, we constructed a simple scatterplot of the item difficulty parameters to help visualize the relative ordering of the ten transitive reasoning items (see Fig. 7.3). We labeled the points in the scatterplot with the item numbers to facilitate interpretation.

```
## Plot item difficulty:
plot(1:10, m1.fixed_items.ordered$difficulty,
xlab = "Item Number", ylab = "Item Difficulty",
main = "Item Difficulty Parameters: \nModel 1",
axes = FALSE, ylim = c(-4.5, 1.5),
```

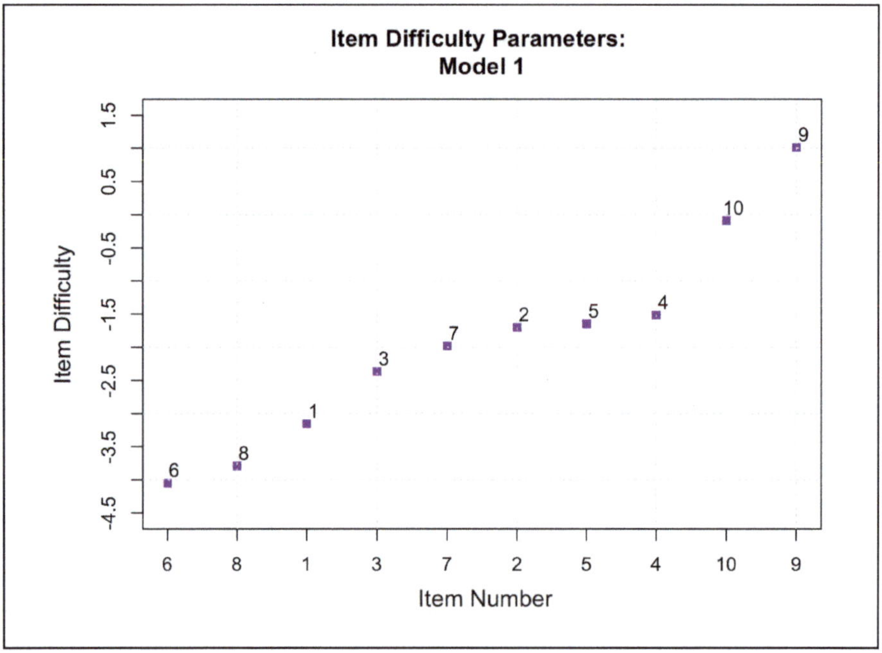

Fig. 7.3 Scatterplot of item difficulty parameters for transitive reasoning items from the Dichotomous Rasch model

```
pch = 15, col = "purple")
axis(1, at = c(1:10), labels = m1.fixed_
items.ordered$item.n)
axis(2, at = seq(-4.5, 1.5, by = .5))
box()
grid()
text((1:10)+.1, m1.fixed_items.ordered$difficulty + .2,
m1.fixed_items.ordered$item.n)
```

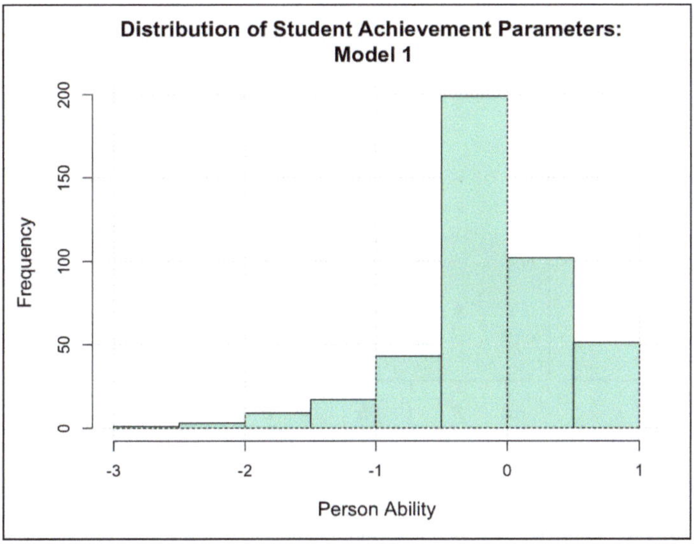

Fig. 7.4 Histogram of student achievement parameters from the transitive reasoning assessment based on the Dichotomous Rasch model

Item 6 was the easiest transitive reasoning task, and item 9 was the most difficult. We will consider details related to individual item characteristics later in this chapter.

We calculated summary statistics on the student locations. From these results, we can see that the average student location was equal to -0.04 logits (*SD* = 0.67). Student locations ranged from -2.62 logits for the student with the lowest level of achievement in transitive reasoning to 0.97 logits for the student with the highest level of achievement in transitive reasoning. Relative to the average item difficulty location, students exhibited a high overall level of achievement in transitive reasoning. The distribution of student achievement is shown in Fig. 7.4.

As a final step in our analysis for model 1, we constructed a Wright Map with the item difficulty and person achievement parameters. We used the WrightMap() function to generate the display (see Fig. 7.5).

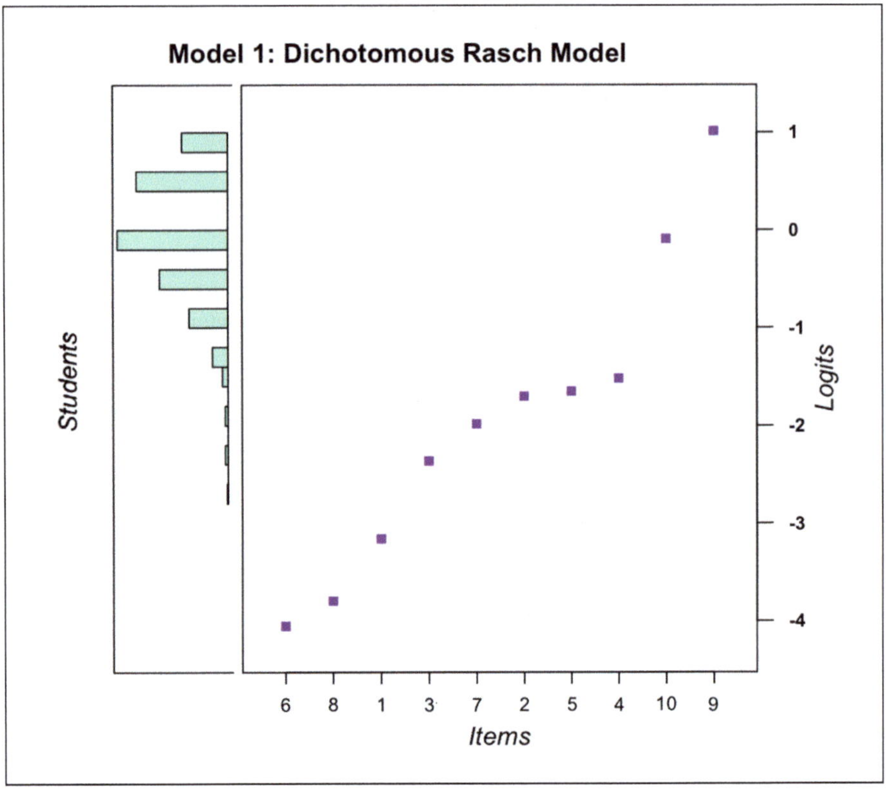

Fig. 7.5 Wright map showing item and student parameter estimates from the transitive reasoning assessment based on the Dichotomous Rasch model

```
wrightMap(thetas = m1.random_students,
thresholds = m1.fixed_items.ordered$difficulty,
show.thr.lab = FALSE,
label.items = m1.fixed_items.ordered$item.n,
thr.sym.pch = 15,
thr.sym.col.fg = "purple",
thr.sym.col.bg = "purple",
dim.color = "aquamarine",
axis.persons = "Students",
dim.names = "",
main.title = "Model 1: Dichotomous Rasch Model")
```

Model 2: Item-Explanatory Model (LLRM)

Our next model is an item-explanatory model in which we incorporate item characteristics into the base model. As we have discussed in earlier chapters, this type of model allows us to examine the degree to which item characteristics provide additional insight into item responses. In the transitive reasoning example, we have one item characteristic that can serve as an explanatory variable: number of objects. Using an item-explanatory model can help us test hypotheses related to the impact of the number of objects involved in a transitive reasoning task on the difficulty of the task. For example, it may be reasonable to predict that more objects are associated with more difficult tasks.

As we saw for the Dichotomous Model and in earlier chapters, specifying explanatory Rasch models in the GLMM framework requires that we include at least one random effect. Following typical practice with the LLRM, we specified the student parameters as random effects and the item covariates (number of objects) as a fixed effect. With this specification, we will focus on the individual item classifications related to the number of objects involved in transitive reasoning tasks. In our data, the tasks included either three or four objects. Other variations on item-explanatory models may include different specifications of these effects.

We estimated Model 2 using the glmer function, with a random effect specification for students. We included "n.objects" as a fixed effect, which reflects the number of objects included in each transitive reasoning task. We stored the results in an object named m2.

```
m2 <- glmer(response ~ -1 + n.objects + (1|Student),
family = binomial("logit"),
data = transreas_long.ordered,
control = control)
```

From the model results, we extracted the location parameters for the item covariates—these are the item classifications related to the number of objects. Similar to our previous model, these values reflect easiness levels by default. We multiplied them by -1 to convert them to difficulty parameters. Then, we used the View() function to examine the estimates.

```
# Extract the fixed item covariate estimates:
m2.fixed_items <- data.frame(easiness = fixef(m2))
## Convert easiness to difficulty for item covariates:
m2.fixed_items$difficulty <- m2.fixed_items$easiness * -1
## View the location estimates:
View(m2.fixed_items)
```

Tasks involving 3 objects had a difficulty estimate of -2.42 logits, and those involving 4 objects had a difficulty estimate of 0.47 logits. These values provide evidence to support our hypothesis that additional objects contribute to increased task difficulty in the transitive reasoning assessment. We created a simple plot of the covariate locations to visualize these results (see Fig. 7.6).

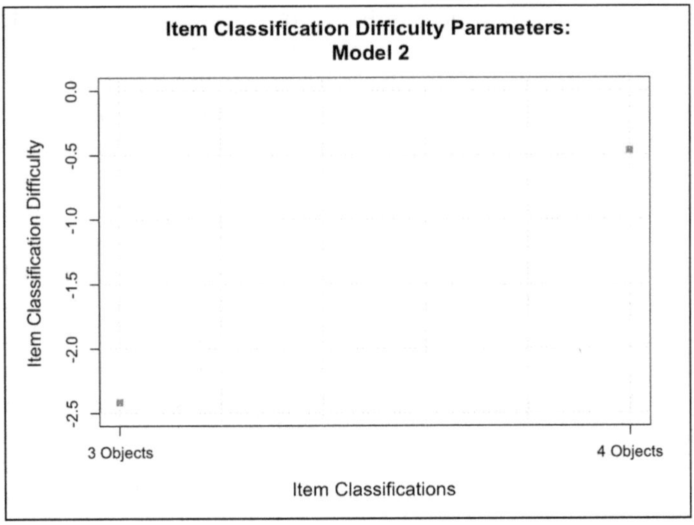

Fig. 7.6 Item covariate parameter estimates from the transitive reasoning assessment based on the LLRM

```
## Create a plot of item covariate difficulty estimates:
graphics.off()
plot(1:2, m2.fixed_items$difficulty,
xlab = "Item Classifications", ylab = "Item Classification
Difficulty",
main = "Item Classification Difficulty Parameters: \nModel
2",
axes = FALSE,
pch = 15,
col = "orchid2",
ylim = c(-2.5, 0))
axis(1, at = c(1:2), labels = c("3 Objects", "4 Objects"))
axis(2, at = seq(-2.5, 0, by = .5))
box()
grid()
```

Next, we extracted student location parameters. As we did for Model 1, we specified students as a random parameter. Accordingly, we do not focus on individual student location estimates here, but rather examine the overall distribution using a histogram (see Fig. 7.7).

```
# Extract the random student parameters:
random <- coef(m2)
m2.random_students <- random$Student[, 1]
```

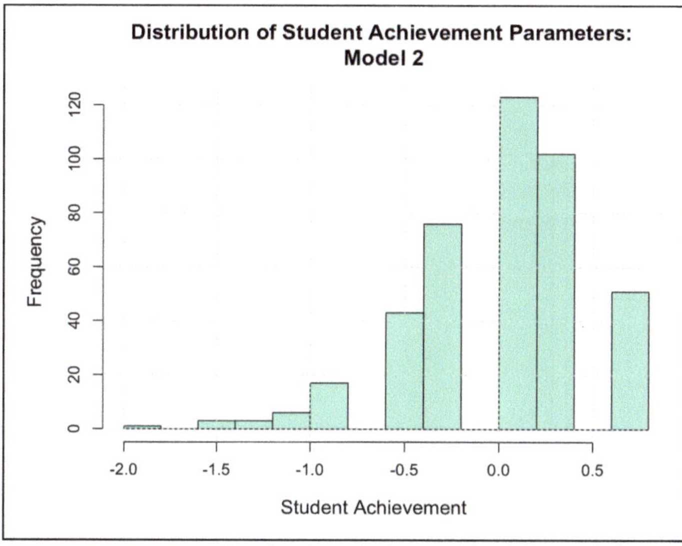

Fig. 7.7 Histogram of student achievement parameter estimates from the transitive reasoning assessment based on the LLRM

We can see some differences in the distribution of student achievement parameters between Model 1 (Fig. 7.4) and Model 2 (Fig. 7.7). Whereas in Model 1, we modeled individual items, Model 2 only included item covariates. Accordingly, there is less distinction between individual students in the parameter estimates from Model 2.

Finally, we constructed a Wright Map with the random student locations and fixed item classification difficulty parameters (see Fig. 7.8).

```
## Plot Wright Map for Model 2:
graphics.off()
wrightMap(thetas=m2.random_students,
thresholds=m2.fixed_items$difficulty,
show.thr.lab = FALSE,
label.items = c("3 Objects", "4 Objects"),
thr.sym.pch = 15,
thr.sym.col.fg = "purple",
thr.sym.col.bg = "purple",
dim.color = "aquamarine",
axis.persons = "Students",
dim.names = "",
main.title = "Model 2: LLRM")
```

Model 3: Person and Item Explanatory Model

The third model is a person-explanatory model in which we included person characteristics alongside item characteristics. This type of model allows us to examine

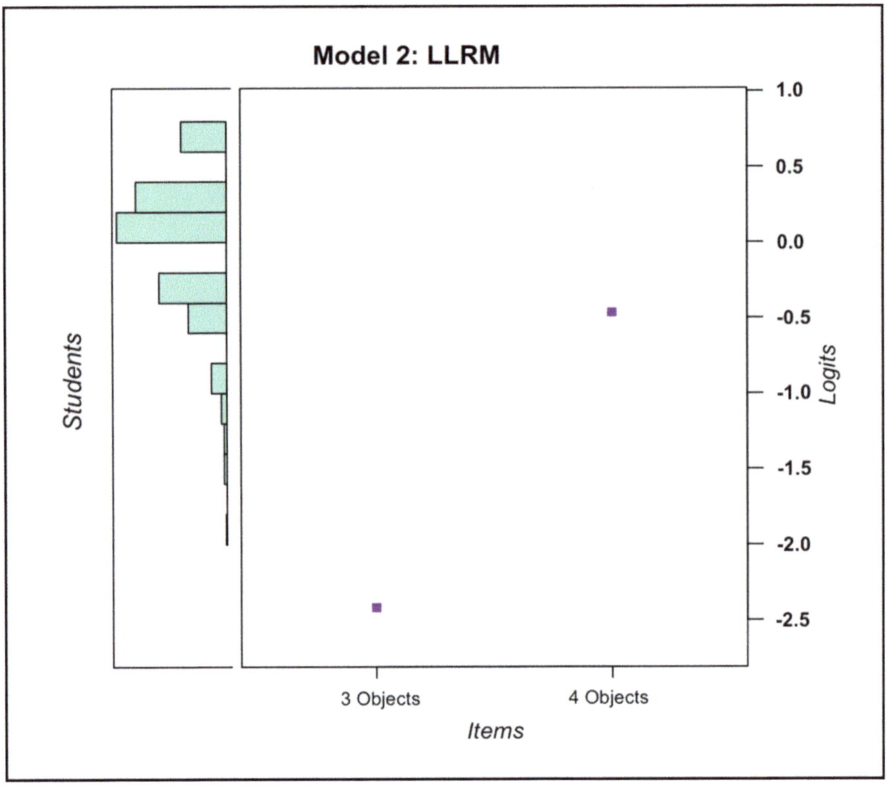

Fig. 7.8 Wright map showing item and student achievement parameter estimates from the transitive reasoning assessment based on the LLRM

the degree to which person characteristics contribute to item responses. In the transitive reasoning example, we have one person characteristic that can serve as an explanatory variable: grade level. Using a person-explanatory model can help us test hypotheses related to the impact of student grade level on the difficulty of transitive reasoning tests. For example, it may be reasonable to assume that task difficulty decreases as student grade level increases

As noted earlier, we need to include at least one random effect in our explanatory model. For continuity with our previous examples, we specified the student location parameters as random effects. We also specified the item characteristic (number of items) as a random effect. We specified student grade level as a fixed effect. This specification allowed us to focus on student grade level as an explanatory variable. Other variations on person and item-explanatory models may include different specifications of these effects.

We estimated Model 3 using the glmer function, with a random effect specification for students (1|Student), a random effect specification for the number of objects

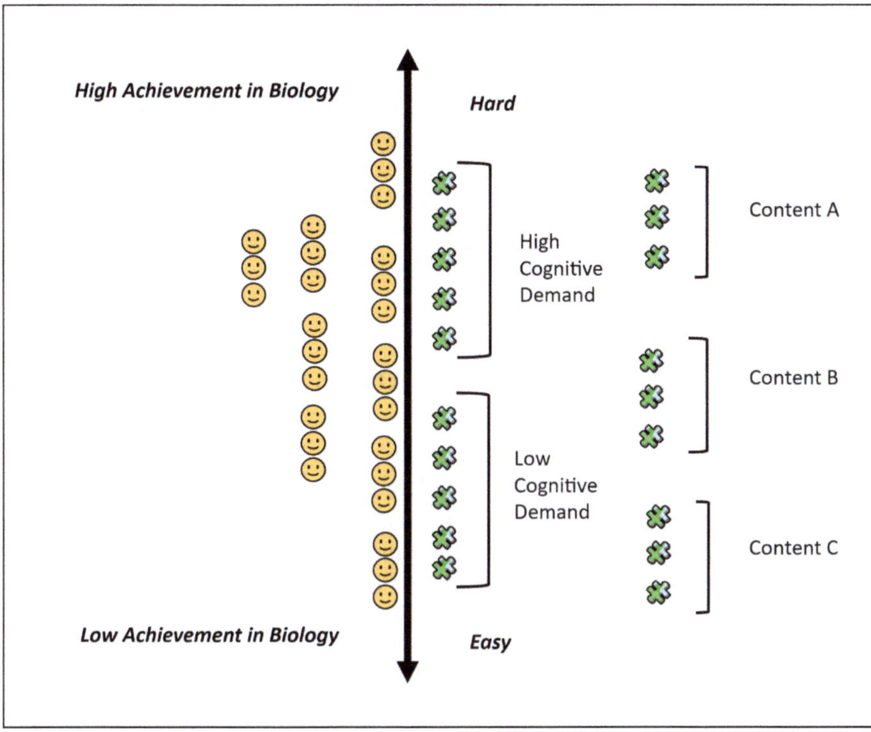

Fig. 7.9 Construct map for biology exam

(1|n.objects), and a fixed effect specification for student grade level (grade.f). We stored the results in an object named m3.

```
m3 <- glmer(response ~ -1 + (1|Student) +
(1|n.objects) + grade.f,
family = binomial("logit"),
data = transreas_long.ordered,
control = control)
```

The main focus of our analysis with Model 3 is on the impact of the student characteristic (grade level) on item difficulty. Recognizing this, we will proceed to examine the fixed effect estimates for student grade level. We extracted the fixed effect estimates for student grade level from the model object and stored the results in an object called "m3.fixed_students."

```
# Extract the fixed student covariate estimates:
```

```
m3.fixed <- data.frame(easiness = fixef(m3))
m3.fixed_students <- m3.fixed$easiness
```

By default, the covariate effects are reported as easiness parameters such that higher values indicate easier items (i.e., less difficulty). In the context of the transitive reasoning analysis, higher easiness parameters for student grade levels indicate that students responded correctly to transitive reasoning tasks more often. Item easiness generally increased as grade levels progressed from grade 2 to grade 6 as expected.

Summary of Transitive Reasoning Analyses

The previous section included several analyses of the Transitive Reasoning Assessment data using an explanatory Rasch modeling approach. Returning to Table 7.2, these analyses reflect the Measurement Model and Structural Aspects components of the instrument development process. The preliminary analysis using the dichotomous Rasch model allowed us to examine the overall progression of item locations from easy to difficult and consider the item hierarchy with reference to the expected order based on theory or item specifications. For persons, we examined the overall distribution of student achievement estimates. Although we did not have details about individual students beyond general grade level classifications, we considered the overall student distribution with reference to the overall item distribution. We observed that our sample of students found the transitive reasoning items relatively easy—evidenced by relatively high achievement parameters compared to item difficulty parameters.

Reflecting the structural aspect for items, we examined the contribution of item classifications with respect to the number of items (3 or 4) using the LLRM. As expected, the transitive reasoning tasks involving 4 objects were more difficult compared to those involving 3 objects. This finding is congruent with theory regarding transitive reasoning (Bouwmeester & Sijtsma, 2004).

Reflecting the structural aspect for persons, we used the latent regression LLRM to consider the influence of student characteristics on response accuracy. Using grade level as a student covariate, we found that items decreased in difficulty as student grade level increased. We expected this pattern based on developmental theory regarding transitive reasoning (Bouwmeester & Sijtsma, 2004). Overall, the series of analyses with explanatory Rasch models allowed us to examine overall item difficulty, the contribution of item covariates, and the impact of person covariates on response probabilities.

Illustration Two: Biology Exam

Our second illustration uses data from a biology exam to illustrate the five components for instrument development. In this illustration, we focus primarily on item characteristics using a LLRM approach. This section includes a brief overview of the biology exam instrument with respect to the construct, observational design, and

Table 7.4 Components for instrument development applied to the biology exam

Components	Questions	Overall	Items
Construct	What is the construct being measured?	Biology content knowledge	Tasks reflecting lower levels of cognitive demand are expected to be easier to solve correctly.
Observational design	What is the plan for collecting structured responses or observations from persons?	Selected-response items administered to students	Items developed based on biology curriculum and theory about cognitive demand
Scoring rules	How are responses or observations categorized to represent person locations on the latent variable?	Item responses scored for correctness	Items categorized based on biology content domain and cognitive demand
Measurement model	How are person and item responses or observations mapped onto the latent variable?	Dichotomous Rasch Model	LLRM
Structural aspects	What are the relationships examined?	Student achievement and item difficulty	Item covariates estimated and used to examine predicted theoretical implications

scoring rules components. Then, we provide a summary of results from the analyses using explanatory Rasch models that reflect the measurement model and structural components. The R code used in this section is based on the EIRM package (Bulut, 2021). This code demonstrates a slightly different approach to conducting these analyses from the first illustration. Table 7.4 provides an overview of the components for instrument development applied to the biology exam. This assessment includes 25 multiple-choice biology items.

Construct

As summarized in Table 7.5, the biology exam was designed to measure levels of knowledge related to five biology content domains: cells, cellular genetics and heredity, classification and phylogeny, ecology, and theory of evolution. Items were distributed between these content domains to reflect statewide assessment standards for biology. Items were classified in two levels of cognitive demand: level 2 or level 3. Items classified within lower levels of cognitive demand are expected to be easier than those involving higher levels of cognitive demand.

Figure 7.9 provides an example of a construct map that could be used along with the biology exam. The left side of the figure shows the distribution of students who are ordered by achievement level in biology, and the right side of the figure reflects

Table 7.5 Classification of biology Items by content domain and cognitive demand

Content domains	Items	Cognitive demands
Cells	1, 2	Level 2 (Low)
	3, 25	Level 3 (High)
Cellular genetics & heredity	5, 6, 7, 10, 12, 23	Level 2 (Low)
	9	Level 3 (High)
Classification & phylogeny	13, 14, 15, 16, 17	Level 2 (Low)
Ecology	7, 17, 20, 21	Level 2 (Low)
	22, 24	Level 3 (High)
Theory of evolution	4, 19	Level 2 (Low)
	11	Level 3 (High)

Note The structure of content domains is based on the statewide assessment standards for Biology

item-related hypotheses related to cognitive demand and content classification. Our biology exam data do not include student-related covariates, so these are not included in the illustration.

Observational Design

Each of the biology exam items required students to respond to respond to a question or complete a task that reflected biology learning objectives related to one of the five content domains. Student responses were scored as either correct or incorrect according to pre-specified keyed responses. Multiple-choice items were created to define the construct of biology achievement. The 25 items are classified in terms of five content areas, and two levels of cognitive demand (Level 2=skills and concepts, Level 3=strategic thinking). Table 7.5 shows the classification of the biology items.

Scoring Rules

Student responses that indicated a correct understanding of the biology concepts received a score of "1". Those that were incorrect received a score of "0". Students with more-frequent correct scores were interpreted as exhibiting higher levels of biology achievement compared to those with less-frequent correct scores.

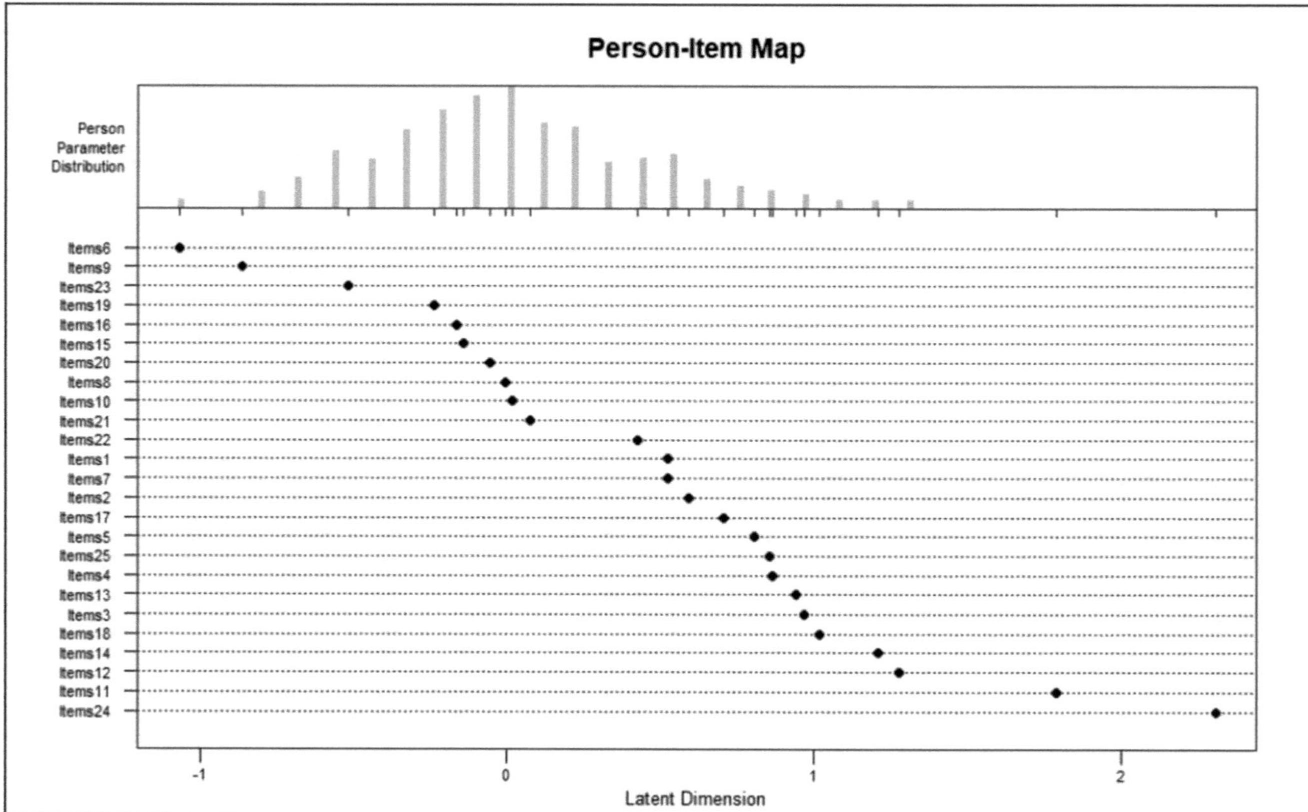

Fig. 7.10 Wright map showing item and student parameter estimates from the biology exam based on the Dichotomous Rasch model

Measurement Model

We analyzed student responses to the biology exam items using a series of models via the EIRM package (Bulut, 2021). We provide an overview of our procedure and results here. Following the same general procedure as with the Transitive Reasoning assessment data, we analyzed the biology exam responses using the dichotomous Rasch model; this model served as a baseline model upon which to build explanatory Rasch models. We used the dichotomous Rasch model to estimate difficulty parameters for the 25 individual biology exam items and achievement parameters for our sample of 573 students. Figure 7.10 shows a Wright Map that illustrates item difficulty and student achievement parameters. Produced using the EIRM package, this figure has a slightly different structure from the Wright Maps that we presented earlier in this chapter. The horizontal axis at the bottom of the figure labeled "Latent Dimension" shows the logit scale; this is the scale on which item and person locations are estimated that reflects the biology achievement construct. The large rectangular panel with dotted lines and black dots shows the item difficulty estimates, with item labels listed along the vertical axis on the left side of the figure. Items are sorted by difficulty from easy at the top of the figure to difficult at the bottom of the figure. For each item, a solid black circle shows the item difficulty parameter on the logit scale. A dotted horizontal line extends from each item label through the plot to help readers map item locations to item labels. At the top of the figure, a histogram shows the distribution of person (student) parameters on the logit scale, where higher bars indicate more students. Based on these results, we can see that there is generally good targeting between the item and person distributions on the biology achievement construct.

Structural Aspects

We applied a series of item-explanatory LLRMs to the biology exam data. Our analyses included LLRMs with different combinations of the item covariates. Model 2 is an LLRM with cognitive demand level as an item covariate; Model 3 is an LLRM with content domain as an item covariate; Model 4 is an LLRM with both cognitive demand level and content domain as item covariates. As we saw for the Transitive Reasoning assessment, these item-explanatory models can help us test hypotheses related to the impact of item classifications on item difficulty. For the biology exam, it is reasonable to predict that items classified in cognitive demand level 3 will be more difficult than those classified in level 2. We did not have specific expectations about the difficulty of items classified within the content domains.

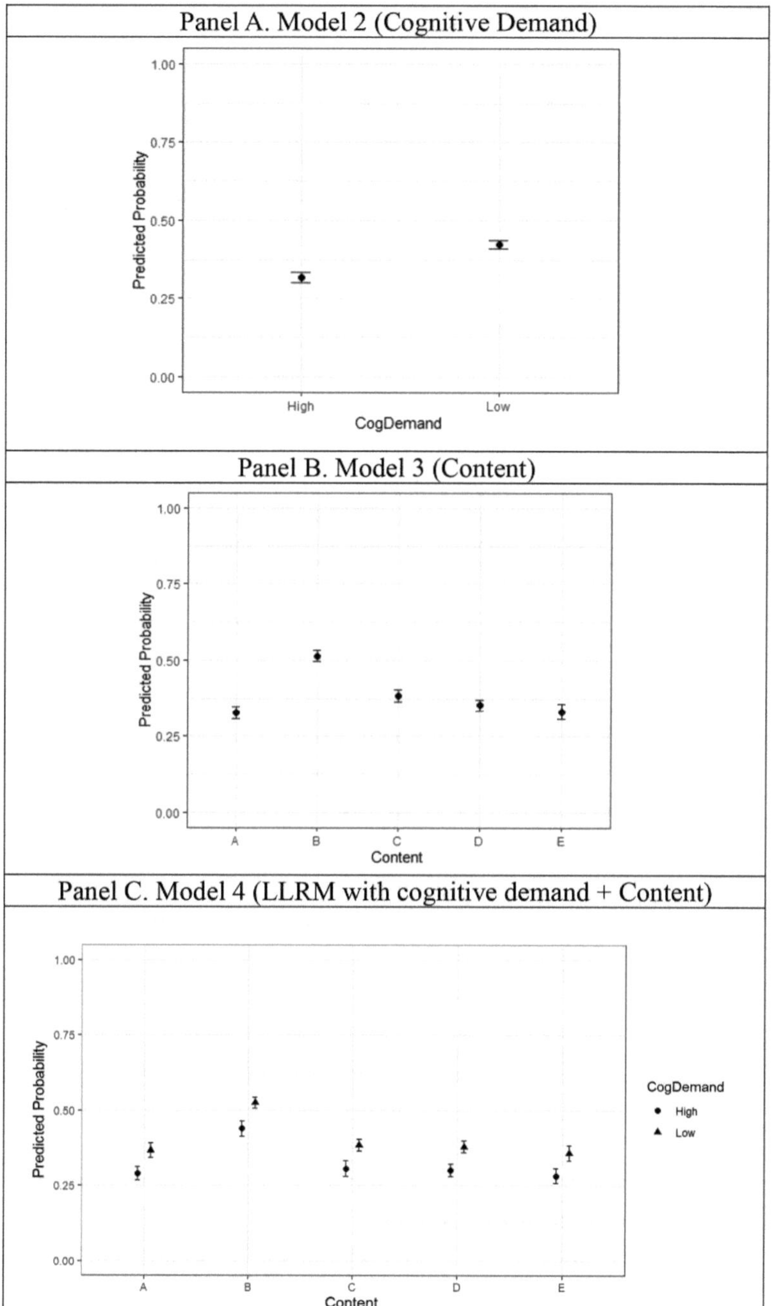

Fig. 7.11 Effects of cognitive demand and content for biology exam

Data Preparation for Biology Exam

The responses to the biology items were analyzed with the EIRM package in R (Bulut, 2021). The first step is to import the data set, and prepare the data for analysis by reshaping the wide form of the data to a long form.

```
# Read in data
rm(list=ls())
library(eirm)
library(dplyr)
library(xlsx)
x <- read.csv("BiologyExam.csv",header=TRUE)
head(x)
```

Next, the Biology Exam data are converted from wide format to long format. The classification of the items by content and cognitive demand is also added at this step.

```
# Convert data to long format
longdata <- melt(x, id.vars=c("Person"), variable.name =
"Item",
value.name = "Response")
# Classify items by cognitive demand
longdata$CogDemand = case_when(longdata$Item %in% c("I1",
"I2","I5","I6","I7",
"I10","I12","I23","I13","I14","I15","I16","I17","I7","I17"
,"I20","I21","I4","I19") ~ "Low",
longdata$Item %in% c("I3", "I25","I9","I22","I24","I11") ~
"High")
# Classify items by content
longdata$Content = case_when(longdata$Item %in%
c("I1","I2","I3","I25") ~ "A",
longdata$Item %in% c("I5","I6","I7","I10","I12","I23","I9")
~ "B",
longdata$Item %in% c("I13","I14","I15","I16","I17") ~ "C",
longdata$Item %in% c("I7","I17","I20","I21","I22","I24","I9")
~ "D",
longdata$Item %in% c("I4","I19","I11") ~ "E")
head(longdata)
```

Model 1: Dichotomous Rasch Model

Next, the EIRM package is used to estimate Dichotomous Rasch model (Model 1), and the variable map is printed as shown in Fig. 7.10.

```
# Rasch model
mod1 <- eirm( "Response ~ -1 + Item + (1|Person)", data =
longdata)
print(mod1, difficulty = TRUE) # To get difficulty parameters
plot(mod1,difficulty = TRUE )
```

Model 2: Item-Explanatory Model (LLRM) with Cognitive Demand
The Linear Logistic Rasch Model is estimated next with cognitive demand as a covariate. The predicted probabilities are shown in Fig. 7.11. (Panel A). As expected, the items with lower cognitive demand have a higher average predicted probability of success by the students.

```
# LLRM with cognitive demand
mod2 <- eirm( "Response ~ -1 + CogDemand + (1|Person)", data =
longdata)
marginalplot(mod2, predictors = c("CogDemand"))
```

Model 3: Item-Explanatory Model (LLRM) with Item Content
Next, the predicted probability for item content is estimated, and plotted in Fig. 7.11 (Panel B).

```
# LLRM with item content
mod3 <- eirm("Response ~ -1 + Content + (1|Person)", data =
longdata)
marginalplot(mod3, predictors = c("Content"))
```

Model 4: Item-Explanatory Model (LLRM) with Cognitive Demand and Item Content
Figure 7.11 (Panel C) shows the predicted probabilities for items as classified by cognitive demand and content. Content B is easiest on average, and the low cognitive demand items are also consistently easier across content areas in biology.

```
# LLRM with CogDemand and Content
mod4 <- eirm( "Response ~ -1 + CogDemand + Content +
(1|Person)", data = longdata)
marginalplot(mod4, predictors = c("Content", "CogDemand"))
```

Summary of Biology Exam Analyses

Figure 7.11 illustrates the item covariate estimates for these models. As shown in Fig. 7.11 (Panel A), items classified within cognitive demand level 3 (high) were more difficult than those classified within cognitive demand level 2 (low). With respect to content domain (Fig. 7.11, Panel B), items classified in the content domains of Cells and Ecology were more difficult than those associated with the other domains. As shown in Fig. 7.11 (Panel C), the relative order of cognitive demand level and content domains persisted when both item classifications were included as explanatory variables. The order of these effects is congruent with our theories about cognitive demand.

Discussion and Summary

In this chapter, we discussed instrument development through the lens of explanatory Rasch models. We proposed five interconnected components for developing measurement tools: Construct, Observational Design, Scoring Rules, Measurement Model, and Structural Aspects. Each component supports an organized, theory-backed approach to assessment creation, factoring in both item-related (e.g., difficulty) and person-related (e.g., demographic characteristics) variables. Each of the components can be briefly described as follows:

1. Construct: The foundational element where researchers define the concept or latent trait being measured, often represented visually with construct maps. These maps help clarify relationships among test items and person characteristics.
2. Observational Design: This involves planning data collection through test items or structured observations aligned with the construct's characteristics.
3. Scoring Rules: These rules convert observations into ordinal data that reflect achievement or ability levels, helping to classify responses along the construct continuum.
4. Measurement Model: The Rasch model translates scored responses into measures on a continuum, supporting consistency in estimating both item difficulty and person ability.
5. Structural Aspects: These involve examining covariates, like item characteristics and demographic factors, to understand their influence on test outcomes.

We provided two illustrative analyses: one on transitive reasoning, which used a dichotomous Rasch model with adjustments for item complexity and grade level, and another on a biology exam where content domains and cognitive demand levels were used as item covariates. Each example demonstrated how explanatory Rasch models can play a role in improving measurement accuracy and guiding revisions by identifying misalignments between observed and expected results. We concluded the chapter by emphasizing the importance of theory-driven and context-sensitive measurement for developing effective assessment instruments.

In summary, explanatory Rasch models should be used to inform each aspect of the item and test development process. There is a need for more research to explore how these models can be integrated into the ongoing processes within a broader measurement context.

References

Bates, D., Maechler, M., Bolker, B., & Walker, S. (2024). *lme4: Linear Mixed-Effects Models using Eigen and S4* (Version 1.1–35.5, p. 1.1–35.5) [R]. https://CRAN.R-project.org/package=lme4

Bouwmeester, S., & Sijtsma, K. (2004). Measuring the ability of transitive reasoning, using product and strategy information. *Psychometrika, 69*(1), 123–146. https://doi.org/10.1007/BF02295743

Bulut, O. (2021). *eirm: Explanatory item response modeling for dichotomous and polytomous item responses* (Version 0.3.0) [R]. https://CRAN.R-project.org/package=eirm.

Embretson, S. (2023). Understanding examinees item responses through cognitive modeling of response accuracy and response times. *Large-Scale Assessments in Education, 11*(1), 9. https://doi.org/10.1176/s40536-023-00157-7

Engelhard, G., & Wang, J. (2021). *Rasch models for solving measurement problems: Invariant measurement in the social sciences.* Sage.

Lane, S., Raymond, M. R., & Haladyna, T. M. (Eds.). (2016). *Handbook of test development* (Vol. 2, pp. 3–17). Routledge.

Luecht, R. (2013). Assessment engineering task model maps, task models and templates as a new way to develop and implement test specifications. *Journal of Applied Testing Technology, 1*, 1–37.

Luecht, R. M. (2025). *Assessment engineering in test design: Methods and applications.* Taylor & Francis.

Torres Irribarra, D., & Freund, R. (2014). *Wright Map: IRT item-person map with ConQuest integration* [Computer software]. http://github.com/david-ti/wrightmap

Wilson, M. (2005). *Constructing measures: An item response modeling approach.* Routledge.

Wilson, M. (2023). *Constructing measures: An item response modeling approach* (2nd ed.). Routledge.

Chapter 8
Rating Scale Analysis for Polytomous Explanatory Rasch Models

Assessments with ratings in ordered categories have become ubiquitous in health, biological and social sciences (Andrich, 2011*, p. 571)*

The focus of this chapter is on rating scale analysis for polytomous explanatory Rasch models. Rating scale analysis (Wind, 2023; Wright & Masters, 1982) is a set of analyses focused on evaluating ordinal response scales (e.g., Likert-type scales or achievement scales in scoring rubrics) for evidence of effective psychometric properties. Because it focuses on the response scale, rating scale analysis provides additional insight into the psychometric quality of measurement procedures beyond what can be learned from overall item-level and person-level analyses.

Although it is possible to conduct rating scale analysis with non-Rasch polytomous IRT models (Wind, 2022, 2023), discussions of rating scale functioning have occurred most often in combination with polytomous Rasch models. Polytomous Rasch models are well-suited to rating scale analysis for several reasons. First, the models use adjacent-categories threshold parameters (Mellenbergh, 1995). For example, the Partial Credit Model (PCM; Masters, 2018) defines the ratio of probabilities for a rating in category k and the category just below it (k – 1). Using a log-odds representation, the model can be written as follows:

$$\ln\left[\frac{P_{n(xi=k)}}{P_{n(xi=k-1)}}\right] = \theta_n - \delta_{ik}, \tag{8.1}$$

where θ_n is the location of person n on the logit scale, and δ_{ik} is the location of the threshold between category k and category k – 1 specific to item i. This value represents the location on the logit scale at which there is an equal probability for a response in category k and category k – 1, specific to item i. This adjacent-categories formulation of the threshold facilitates checks for category ordering (Andrich, 2015; Wind, 2022; we discuss ordering in more detail later). The use of adjacent-categories formulations for Rasch model threshold parameters has made threshold ordering a

G. Engelhard and S. A. Wind, *Invariant Measurement with Explanatory Rasch Models in the Human Sciences*, https://doi.org/10.1007/978-3-032-08816-1_8

point of emphasis and discussion in literature related to Rasch models (Adams et al., 2012; Andrich, 2013; Wetzel & Carstensen, 2014).

Second, researchers who use Rasch models are often interested in improving their measurement procedures (Engelhard & Wang, 2020). Rating scale analysis provides a variety of indicators that can inform revisions to measurement procedures. Although rating scale analysis has been discussed in detail in the context of descriptive Rasch models, this topic has not received specific attention with reference to explanatory Rasch models. With this chapter, we hope to provide some preliminary ideas and guidance related to how rating scale analysis can be conceptualized for explanatory Rach models.

The remainder of this chapter is organized as follows. In the next section, we introduce the illustrative data that we will use throughout the chapter. Then, we review methods for estimating polytomous Rasch models within a Generalized Linear Mixed Modeling (GLMM) framework. We illustrate how polytomous Rasch models can be estimated in the EIRM package (Bulut, 2021) to obtain threshold estimates necessary for rating scale analysis. We demonstrate rating scale analysis techniques using estimates from the PCM. After that, we discuss and illustrate two explanatory Rasch models that facilitate rating scale analysis: an item-explanatory model and a person-explanatory model. We consider how these models provide insight into rating scale functioning related to item and person characteristics. We conclude the chapter with a summary and discussion, highlighting areas for further investigation.

Illustrative Analyses of the CESD Data

This chapter includes illustrative analyses based on responses to the Center for Epidemiological Studies Depression (CESD) scale (Radloff, 1977). The data included in our analyses were simulated to reflect the results from a recent administration of the CESD scale (Donny et al., 2015) for illustrative purposes. Specifically, data were simulated based on parameters reported from the baseline time point in Donny et al. (2015), which were calculated using the Generalized Partial Credit Model (Muraki, 1997). The CESD scale was developed to measure depression using twenty items that describe feelings and behaviors. Participants respond to the items using a frequency scale with four ordered categories to indicate how often they experienced a feeling or exhibited a behavior over the previous week: 1 = *Rarely or none of the time* (less than 1 day); 2 = *Some or a little of the time* (1–2 days); 3 = *Occasionally or a moderate amount of time* (3-4 days); 4 = *Most or all of the time* (5–7 days). Table 8.1 shows the item stems for the CESD. Four of the items (items 4, 8, 12, and 16) required reverse-coding prior to analysis. In our analyses, we recoded the original responses such that the lowest category is equal to zero.

The CESD dataset that we use in this chapter also includes several demographic variables related to the participants. Specifically, our data include participants' self-reported classifications related to gender (1 = Male; 2 = Female), living situation (1 = Live alone; 2 = Live with significant other/kids; 3 = Live with parents; 4 = Live with friends/relatives; 5 = Other), and education level (1 = 8th grade or less, 2 = Some high school; 3 = High School/Grad Equiv.; 4 = Some college/2-year; 5 = 4-year college; 6 = Grad/Prof).

Table 8.1 CESD item stems and classifications

Item number	Item stem	Feelings (F) or actions (A) classification
1	I was bothered by things that usually don't bother me	A
2	I did not feel like eating; my appetite was poor	F
3	I felt I could not cheer up, even with the help of my family or friends	A
4 (R)	I felt that I was just as good as other people	A
5	I had trouble keeping my mind on what I was doing	F
6	I felt depressed	A
7	I felt that everything I did was an effort	A
8 (R)	I felt hopeful about the future	A
9	I thought my life had been a failure	A
10	I felt fearful	A
11	My sleep was restless	F
12 (R)	I was happy	A
13	I talked less than usual	F
14	I felt lonely	A
15	People were unfriendly	A
16 (R)	I enjoyed life	A
17	I had crying spells	F
18	I felt sad	F
19	I felt that people dislike me	F
20	I could not get "going"	F

Note Items 4, 8, 12, and 16 require reverse-coding (R) prior to analysis

We prepared the R environment for analyses by loading the EIRM package (Bulut, 2021) and the TAM package (Robitzsch et al., 2020). Then, we imported the data as we have done throughout this book.

```
## Load eirm package
library(eirm)
## Load TAM package
library(TAM)
## Import data:
setwd("~/Documents/Wind/GE SW Explanatory Models Book/rating
scale analysis chapter")
cesd <- read.csv("CESD.csv")
```

Estimating Polytomous Rasch Models in the GLMM Framework

Because they use a binomial distribution (see Chapter 2), GLMM formulations of Rasch models require dichotomous dependent variables. Accordingly, it is necessary to recode polytomous item responses to dichotomous variables to estimate polytomous Rasch models in this framework. Bulut et al. (2021) proposed an approach to recoding ordinal polytomous item responses for analyses with explanatory Rasch models. We illustrate this approach in Table 8.2. As presented by Bulut et al., the recoding approach involves creating $k - 1$ "pseudo-dichotomous" response variables from an ordinal response scale with k categories. Bulut et al. refer to these re-coded response variables as "polycategory" variables.

Similar to dummy coding in regression analyses (Fox, 2016), these variables represent adjacent-categories combinations of the original ordinal response categories. In the case of the CESD scale, whose items include a four-category ordinal response scale ($x = 0, 1, 2, 3$), the recoding procedure results in three pseudo-dichotomous response variables that represent dichotomizations of each pair of adjacent response categories (0–1; 1–2; and 2–3). For each pseudo-dichotomous variable, a value of 1 indicates a response in the higher category within the pair, and a value of 0 indicates a response in the lower category. The pseudo-dichotomous variables are coded as missing data (i.e., "NA") when the original response is not included in either category represented by the recoded variable.

Using this approach, an original response in category 0 is represented using a score of 0 on the first pseudo-dichotomous response variable (0-1) and missing values on the second (1-2) and third (2-3) pseudo-dichotomous response variables. An original response in category 1 is represented with a value of 1 for the first pseudo-dichotomous response variable (0-1), a value of 0 for the second pseudo-dichotomous response variable (1-2), and a missing value for the third pseudo-dichotomous response variable (2-3). An original response in category 2 is represented with a missing value for the first pseudo-dichotomous response variable (0-1), a value of 1 for the second pseudo-dichotomous response variable (1-2), and a value of 0 for the third pseudo-dichotomous response variable. Finally, an original response in category 3 is represented with missing values for the first two pseudo-dichotomous response variables (0-1 and 1-2), and a value of 1 for the third pseudo-dichotomous

Table 8.2 Illustration of polytomous recoding for GLMM estimation

Original response	Pseudo-dichotomous response variables (i.e., thresholds)		
	(0–1)	(1–2)	(2–3)
0	0	NA	NA
1	1	0	NA
2	NA	1	0
3	NA	NA	1

response variable (2-3). With this recoding scheme, the original polytomous item response data are re-coded to dichotomous variables that can be modeled using a GLMM approach.

The EIRM package (Bulut, 2021) includes the "polyreformat()" function that facilitates this recoding process for ordinal polytomous data stored in long format. The code below shows how we re-shaped the CESD data to long format, such that each row in the long-format dataset represent a unique person-item combination. Then, we applied the recoding function.

```
## Reshape data to long format:
cesd_long <- reshape(data = cesd,
direction = "long",
varying = 5:24,
timevar = "item",
v.names = "response",
idvar = "id")
## Re-code polytomous responses to category-specific vari-
ables:
cesd_long_poly <- polyreformat(data = cesd_long,
id.var = c("id", "gender", "living", "education"),
var.name = "item",
val.name = "response")
```

The resulting dataset includes item responses to the original CESD scale (labeled "response"), as well as recoded responses to each of the pseudo-dichotomous response variables for each item. The demographic variables are also included in the long-format data. Item-category combinations that make up the pseudo-dichotomous response variables are listed in the variable labeled "polyitem" using the item number followed by "cat_1" to represent the first pair of categories, "cat_2" to represent the second pair of categories, and "cat_3" to represent the third pair of categories in the CESD response scale. Dichotomous responses are stored in the "polyresponse" variable.

As shown in Fig. 8.1, if we sort the data by item, we can see the structure of the recoded data. Each participant's response to each item is represented by three unique rows that represent the three pseudo-dichotomous response variables. For example, participant 1 responded in category 1 for item 1. This response is represented using a value of 1 on polyitem 1.cat_1, a score of 0 on polyitem 1.cat_2, and a missing value on polyitem 1.cat_3.

In addition to dichotomizing the polytomous responses, we also need to change the classification of the item label variable to a factor type so that we can estimate models using EIRM package functions. We created a factor version of the item label variable and added it to the recoded CESD dataset.

Filter

	id	gender	living	education	item	response	polycategory	polyresponse	polyitem
1	1	2	1	4	1	1	cat_1	1	1.cat_1
16781	1	2	1	4	1	1	cat_2	0	1.cat_2
33561	1	2	1	4	1	1	cat_3	NA	1.cat_3
2	2	2	2	4	1	2	cat_1	NA	1.cat_1
16782	2	2	2	4	1	2	cat_2	1	1.cat_2
33562	2	2	2	4	1	2	cat_3	0	1.cat_3
3	3	2	3	3	1	0	cat_1	0	1.cat_1
16783	3	2	3	3	1	0	cat_2	NA	1.cat_2
33563	3	2	3	3	1	0	cat_3	NA	1.cat_3

Fig. 8.1 Illustration of recoded polytomous data using the EIRM package

```
## Change the item variable to factor type:
cesd_long_poly$item.f <- as.factor(cesd_long_poly$item)
```

Next, we will apply the descriptive PCM to our re-coded data using the eirm() function with the polyresponse variable as the dependent variable. Independent variables include the factor version of the item label ("item.f") and the participant identification variable ("id"). To represent the item-specific thresholds in the PCM, we included an interaction between the item and the response category in the formula.

```
## Estimate the PCM
pcm <- eirm(formula = "polyresponse ~ -1 + item.f +
item.f:polycategory + (1|id)",
data = cesd_long_poly)
```

Because we are focusing on rating scale analysis, the item-specific adjacent-category threshold parameters are the focal point for our analyses. We used the following code to create a matrix of item-specific adjacent-category threshold parameters. We multiplied the values by -1 to transform the parameters from the default "easiness" values to reflect difficulty, and stored the resulting values in an object called "pcm.pars".

```
# Create a matrix with item-specific threshold difficulty
estimates:
n.items <- 20
n.thresholds <- 3
pcm.pars <- matrix(data = NA, nrow = n.items, ncol =
n.thresholds)
for(threshold.number in 1:n.thresholds){
```

```
if(threshold.number == 1){
pcm.pars[, threshold.number] <- -1*pcm$parameters[1:n.items,
"Easiness"]
}
if(threshold.number > 1){
pcm.pars[ , threshold.number] <- -1*pcm$parameters[1:n.items,
"Easiness"]-pcm$parameters[(n.items * (threshold.number -
1) + 1):(n.items * threshold.number), "Easiness"]
}
}
View(pcm.pars)
```

The pcm.pars object includes one row for each item in our CESD dataset, with columns that represent the adjacent-category thresholds (labeled "t1", "t2", and "t3") specific to each item. We can now investigate these parameters from the perspective of rating scale analysis.

Our analyses will focus on three major indicators of rating scale functioning: threshold ordering, category precision, and category comparability. Adapted from Wind (2022), Table 8.3 lists the three indicators using corresponding underlying questions that reflect the purpose of their corresponding analyses along with major sources of evidence that can be extracted from polytomous Rasch models, including explanatory Rasch models. We demonstrate these analyses with the CESD data using the descriptive PCM estimated in eirm. These procedures provide a foundation for similar analyses using explanatory versions of the PCM later in this chapter.

Category Ordering

Category ordering refers to the degree to which participant responses in ordinal response categories reflect the expected order based on the researcher's theoretical understanding of the construct. For example, if the categories are ordered as expected for the CESD instrument, responses in lower rating scale categories (e.g., rarely) should reflect less severe depression, while those in higher categories (e.g., often) should reflect more-severe depression. Empirical tests to evaluate category ordering provide researchers with insight related to the degree to which participant interpretation and use of response categories matches their expectations. Evidence of disordering can provide guidance for revising scale category labels or descriptions, revising the structure of a rating scale, or facilitate further investigations of the construct with respect to its progression. Various tools are available with which to evaluate category ordering. As shown in Table 8.3, we recommend three relatively simple techniques, which include two numeric checks and one graphical approach.

The first technique for evaluating category ordering involves calculating simple descriptive statistics on person location estimates (θ) within rating scale categories for each item. Researchers can gain valuable insight into category ordering by investigating the relationship between how participants respond within categories for an

Table 8.3 Indicators of rating scale functioning

Rating Scale Functioning Indicator	Underlying Question	Sources of Evidence
Category Ordering	To what extent do responses in lower and higher categories reflect lower and higher levels of the construct?	• Average person location estimates (θ) within response categories • Relative order of threshold estimates • Graphical displays of category probabilities
Category Precision	To what extent do individual response categories reflect distinct levels of the construct?	• Distance between adjacent threshold estimates • Graphical displays of category probabilities
Category Comparability	To what extent do the response categories have a consistent interpretation between elements of the assessment procedure (e.g., individual items, item classifications, person subgroups)?	• Category ordering and precision specific to individual assessment elements

item of interest and their overall location estimates. Specifically, researchers can calculate the average person location among participants who responded in each category of a selected item. Within items, non-decreasing average person locations as categories move from low to high provides support for an ordinal interpretation of response categories. The code below demonstrates one approach to this analysis for the items in the CESD scale. Our analysis involved several steps, including saving the person location estimates from the PCM in a data frame object, creating an empty matrix in which to store item-specific results, and using a for-loop to add the results to the matrix.

```
## Average person location estimates within categories
### Save person location estimates in a data frame:
thetas <- unlist(pcm$persons$id)
person.locations <- cbind.data.frame(cesd$id, thetas)
names(person.locations) <- c("id", "theta")
### Set up matrix for results:
n.thresholds <- 3
n.items <- 20
cesd.responses <- subset(cesd, select = -c(id, gender,
living, education))
category_thetas <- matrix(data = NA, nrow = n.items, ncol =
n.thresholds + 1)
```

```
### Use a for-loop to add the results to the matrix:
for(item.number in 1:n.items){
item    <-    cbind.data.frame(cesd$id,    cesd.responses[,
item.number])
names(item) <- c("id", "resp")
cat.0 <- subset(item, item$resp == 0)
cat.1 <- subset(item, item$resp == 1)
cat.2 <- subset(item, item$resp == 2)
cat.3 <- subset(item, item$resp == 3)
merged.cat.0 <- merge(cat.0, person.locations, by = "id")
category_thetas[item.number, 1] <- mean(merged.cat.0$theta)
merged.cat.1 <- merge(cat.1, person.locations, by = "id")
category_thetas[item.number, 2] <- mean(merged.cat.1$theta)
merged.cat.2 <- merge(cat.2, person.locations, by = "id")
category_thetas[item.number, 3] <- mean(merged.cat.2$theta)
merged.cat.3 <- merge(cat.3, person.locations, by = "id")
category_thetas[item.number, 4] <- mean(merged.cat.3$theta)
```

```
}
### Label the results:
category_thetas <- cbind.data.frame(colnames(cesd.responses),
category_thetas)
names(category_thetas) <- c("item", "x = 0", "x = 1", "x = 2",
"x = 3")
### View the results:
View(category_thetas)
```

Table 8.4 shows the results for the CESD items. In the CESD dataset, we observed the expected progression of average person locations for all items. This is one source of evidence related to category ordering that we can use in combination with other results.

The second check for category ordering involves evaluating threshold estimates for evidence of the expected ordering. Specifically, researchers can evaluate adjacent-categories thresholds obtained from applications of polytomous measurement models for evidence that the threshold estimates are non-decreasing as their associated rating scale categories progress from low to high. In the case of the CESD example, estimates of the three adjacent-categories thresholds for the four-category rating scale thresholds for each item (i.e., τ_{i1}, τ_{i2}, and τ_{i3}) are expected to progress such that $\tau_{i1} \leq \tau_{i2} \leq \tau_{i3}$. We estimated item-specific threshold values for each item in the CESD dataset earlier in this chapter. The following code uses those values to evaluate ordering for each pair of categories for each item, resulting in a data frame with "true" or "false" values that reflect expected or unexpected ordering, respectively for each pair of adjacent thresholds. We also added an overall test for any disordering associated with an item in a column labeled "any disorder."

Table 8.4 Average person location estimate (θ) within response categories for the CESD dataset

Item Number	Average Person Location Estimate (θ) Among Participants Who Responded Within Rating Scale Categories			
	x=0	*x*=1	*x*=2	*x*=3
1	-0.14	-0.02	0.15	0.40
2	-0.13	0.05	0.20	0.31
3	-0.11	0.09	0.13	0.38
4	-0.11	0.05	0.15	0.27
5	-0.17	0.02	0.20	0.44
6	-0.13	0.04	0.20	0.37
7	-0.14	0.04	0.15	0.38
8	-0.12	0.03	0.09	0.26
9	-0.10	0.07	0.14	0.32
10	-0.12	0.04	0.20	0.33
11	-0.13	0.06	0.23	0.25
12	-0.11	0.00	0.07	0.18
13	-0.13	0.00	0.20	0.34
14	-0.12	0.07	0.20	0.35
15	-0.12	0.02	0.17	0.30
16	-0.10	-0.02	0.11	0.20
17	-0.09	0.09	0.16	0.29
18	-0.15	0.05	0.19	0.36
19	-0.12	0.05	0.16	0.33
20	-0.14	0.04	0.18	0.36

```
## Check threshold ordering:
t1_t2 <- pcm.pars[, 2] <= pcm.pars[, 1]
t2_t3 <- pcm.pars[, 2] <= pcm.pars[, 3]
threshold.order.check <- cbind.data.frame(t1_t2, t2_t3)
threshold.order.check$any_disorder <- threshold.order.check$t1_
t2 == FALSE | threshold.order.check$t2_t3 == FALSE
View(threshold.order.check)
```

Table 8.5 shows the threshold ordering results for the CESD items. Depending on the purpose of the category ordering analysis, researchers may wish to evaluate the magnitude of disordering by incorporating standard errors or significance tests. For our current exploratory purposes, a simple ordering comparison is sufficient.

Threshold comparisons indicated disordering for several CESD items. We observed disordering between the lower two thresholds for the following items: 2, 3, 4, 6, 8, 9, 10, 12, 13, 14, 16, 18, and 19. We observed disordering between the second and third thresholds for items 9 and 11. Together, these results indicate some

Table 8.5 Threshold ordering tests for the CESD items

Item Number	$\tau_1 \leq \tau_2$	$\tau_2 \leq \tau_3$	Any Disordering
1	TRUE	TRUE	No
2	FALSE	TRUE	Yes
3	FALSE	TRUE	Yes
4	FALSE	TRUE	Yes
5	TRUE	TRUE	No
6	FALSE	TRUE	Yes
7	TRUE	TRUE	No
8	FALSE	TRUE	Yes
9	FALSE	FALSE	Yes
10	FALSE	TRUE	Yes
11	TRUE	FALSE	Yes
12	FALSE	TRUE	Yes
13	FALSE	TRUE	Yes
14	FALSE	TRUE	Yes
15	TRUE	TRUE	No
16	FALSE	TRUE	Yes
17	FALSE	TRUE	Yes
18	TRUE	TRUE	No
19	FALSE	TRUE	Yes
20	TRUE	TRUE	No

challenges with rating scale category ordering that particularly affected the lower response categories in the CESD rating scale. These results likely reflect the imperfect targeting between participants and items in this CESD administration, where participants reported relatively low overall levels of depression. As a result, there may have been some ambiguity in distinctions between the categories that reflect infrequent depressive behaviors.

The final indicator of category ordering involves examining visualizations of category response probabilities specific to individual items. Specifically, we recommend examining graphical displays of category probabilities (i.e., category probability curves) alongside numeric checks for category ordering. As shown in Fig. 8.2, these plots illustrate the probability for a response in each observed rating scale category (y-axis) conditional on participant location estimates (θ; x-axis), where separate lines reflect the rating scale categories. With the descriptive PCM, separate plots are constructed for individual items. Visual inspection of these plots for individual items can provide additional insight into the nature of category ordering and disordering to further inform the interpretation and use of model results.

To the best of our knowledge, it is not straightforward to generate these visualizations using EIRM package output. As a result, we will use the TAM package (Robitzsch et al., 2020) to generate them to support our rating scale analyses. The

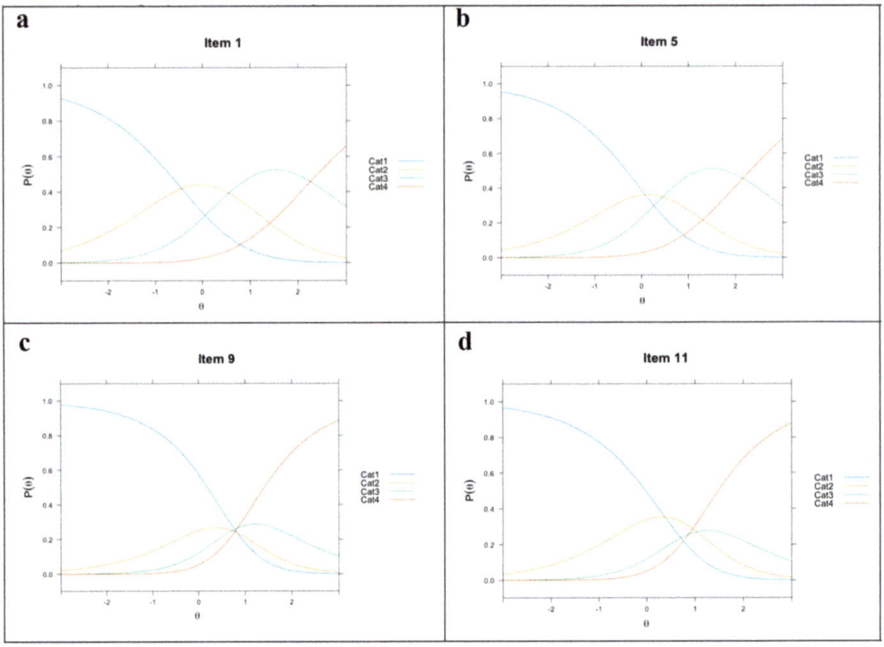

Fig. 8.2 Plots of category probabilities for selected CESD items

following code applies the descriptive PCM to the CESD dataset and then generates plots of category probabilities for each item.

```
# Plots of category probability curves using TAM:
## First, we need to estimate the model using TAM:
### Re-name columns in the response matrix for nicer plot
titles:
names(cesd.responses) <- c(1:n.items)
### Specify the design matrix for the model:
design.matrix <- designMatrices(resp=cesd.responses, model-
type="PCM", constraint = "items")$A
### Run the PCM using the design matrix
PCM.CESD  <-  tam.jml(cesd.responses,  A  =  design.matrix,
constraint = "items",
control=list(maxiter=500), version=2)
## Generate plots of category probabilities
plot(PCM.CESD, type="items")
```

This code produces plots similar to those shown in Fig. 8.2. We selected four CESD items to illustrate different patterns with respect to category ordering. For item 1 (Fig. 8.2A), the plot indicates expected category ordering, where the probabilities for responding in each of the four categories are ordered as expected as participant locations progress from low to high. For Item 5 (Fig. 8.2B), we also observed expected category ordering, although the pattern of response probabilities is different (discussed further later in this chapter). For Item 8 (Fig. 8.2C) and Item 11 (Fig. 8.2D), the plots indicate category disordering at the lower or higher end of the rating scale, respectively.

Category Precision

Category precision refers to the degree to which individual response categories provide unique information about participants with respect to the construct. Category precision indicators help researchers evaluate whether the length of the rating scale (i.e., the number of categories) is sufficient to distinguish between participants with meaningful differences on the construct. For example, in the case of the CESD instrument, evidence of category precision would indicate that the four levels of frequency reflected in the response categories are sufficient to identify participants with meaningfully distinct levels of depression.

We recommend using numeric and graphical checks for category precision, both of which can be obtained using measurement models. For numeric evidence of category precision, researchers can calculate the distance between pairs of adjacent-categories threshold parameters. Whereas distances that are very small may indicate that participants did not easily distinguish between a pair of categories, distances that are very large may indicate that additional levels of distinction (i.e., more categories) may be needed to fully capture the range of the construct. Critical values for establishing a minimum and maximum distance between adjacent thresholds are difficult to establish for general purposes. This difficulty arises because distances between categories are sensitive to many factors including but not limited to the number of categories in the rating scale, the distribution and range of participant and item locations, targeting between participants and items, the nature of the construct, among others.

These considerations notwithstanding and recognizing the need for some guidance, Linacre (2002) suggested a procedure for identifying a minimum distance between adjacent threshold values in rating scale category analysis. His recommendation was specifically targeted to measurement procedures in which it is appropriate to interpret rating scale categories a set of dichotomous items, such as a developmental scale. In this case, he suggested that one can calculate adjacent-categories thresholds using:

$$\tau = \ln\left(\frac{x}{(m-x)+1}\right) \tag{8.2}$$

where *ln* is the natural logarithm, x is the category number, and m is the number of thresholds for the rating scale (i.e., the number of categories in the rating scale minus one). After finding the threshold value for each pair of adjacent categories, one can calculate the distance between them as a guideline for the minimum distance between thresholds.

We can consider this approach for the CESD scale, which has four response categories ($x = 0, 1, 2, 3$). Using Equation 8.2, the threshold values are defined as:

$\tau_1 = ln\ (1/((3\text{-}1)+1)) = -1.10$

$\tau_2 = \ln\ (2/((3\text{-}2)+1)) = 0$

$\tau_3 = \ln\ (3/((3\text{-}3)+1)) = 1.10$

With these values, the absolute value of the recommended minimum distance between categories is 1.10 logits, based on $|\tau_2 - \tau_1|$ and $|\tau_3 - \tau_2|$.

Although this approach is useful for interpreting distances between categories, we emphasize that the resulting values should be interpreted only as a point of reference. Additional information specific to each unique measurement context is critical to determining whether rating scale categories are sufficiently distinct for the intended interpretation and use of the instrument.

In addition to the distance between numeric threshold estimates, researchers can also examine plots of category probabilities (e.g., Fig. 8.2) for evidence related to category precision. When category precision is of interest, researchers can consider the degree to which each category has a distinct peak (i.e., is modal)—indicating that there is a unique range of the construct at which it is the most likely response. Non-modal categories may not provide unique information about participants with respect to the construct.

For the CESD, we observed non-modality for several items, as illustrated in Fig. 8.2. These results suggest that fewer levels of frequency may have been sufficient to capture differences in depressive behaviors in our sample.

Category Comparability

Finally, category comparability refers to the degree to which rating scale categories function in a similar way between elements of an assessment procedure, such as between items, groups of items, or groups of participants. The descriptive PCM allows researchers to evaluate category comparability between items because it provides item-specific threshold estimates. As we will see in the following sections, explanatory Rasch models facilitate category comparability analyses with respect to item-related and person-related covariates.

Rating Scale Analysis with Explanatory Rasch Models

It is also possible to examine rating scale functioning as it relates to item and person covariates using polytomous explanatory Rasch models. Specifically, researchers can specify polytomous explanatory Rasch models such that the rating scale category threshold parameter varies between levels of explanatory variables, such as item or person classifications. With this approach, researchers can evaluate rating scale functioning as it relates to these covariates using methods similar to those from descriptive Rasch models. In the following sections, we demonstrate rating scale analysis related to item covariates and person covariates using item-explanatory and person-explanatory Rasch models.

We did not generate visualizations of rating scale category probabilities for these models because, to the best of our knowledge, they cannot be directly generated using the EIRM package. Nevertheless, the numeric indicators of rating scale functioning provide insight into category ordering and precision for these models.

Rating Scale Analysis with Item-Explanatory Rasch Models

Rating scale analysis with item-explanatory Rasch models involves examining rating scale functioning at the level of item covariates. To illustrate this approach, we will use an item-explanatory polytomous Rasch model to examine differences in rating scale functioning between subsets of the CESD items. This model can be described as a polytomous version of the Linear Logistic Rasch Model that we have discussed in earlier chapters.

As shown in Table 8.1 earlier in this chapter, we classified each of the CESD items based on whether they reflect feelings (F) or actions (A) based on our interpretation of the stems. These classifications served as the item-explanatory covariate in our rating scale analysis. Using the code below, we classified items within feeling or action categories and saved the classifications as a new variable in the long format re-coded version of the data. We labeled items associated with feelings using “F” and those associated with items using “A”.

```
# Add item classifications:
feeling.items <- c(2, 5, 11, 13, 17, 18, 19, 20)
cesd_long_poly$feeling[cesd_long_poly$item          %in%
feeling.items] <- "F"
cesd_long_poly$feeling[(cesd_long_poly$item         %in%
feeling.items) == FALSE] <- "A"
```

In EIRM, we can specify the equation for the item-explanatory model using the following code:

```
lltm_pcm <- eirm(formula = "polyresponse ~ -1 + feeling +
feeling:polycategory + (1|id)", data = cesd_long_poly)
```

Our equation includes an interaction between item classifications (“feeling”) and the rating scale thresholds (“polycategory”). This specification results in rating scale category threshold estimates that are specific to each item classification. We can extract these results from the model and store them in a matrix using the following code. We will use these threshold values in our rating scale analysis.

```
# Extract threshold parameters:
## Create a matrix with item-classification-specific
threshold difficulty estimates:
n.item.groups <- 2
n.thresholds <- 3
lltm_pcm.pars <- matrix(data = NA, nrow = n.item.groups, ncol
= n.thresholds)
for(threshold.number in 1:n.thresholds){
if(threshold.number == 1){
lltm_pcm.pars[ , threshold.number] <- -1*lltm_
pcm$parameters[1:n.item.groups, "Easiness"]
}
if(threshold.number > 1){
lltm_pcm.pars[ , threshold.number] <- -1*lltm_
pcm$parameters[1:n.item.groups, "Easiness"]-lltm_
pcm$parameters[(n.item.groups * (threshold.number - 1) +
1):(n.item.groups * threshold.number), "Easiness"]
}
}
View(lltm_pcm.pars)
```

Rating Scale Category Ordering

We can evaluate rating scale category ordering within each of the item classifications using similar methods to those demonstrated earlier with the descriptive PCM. Reflecting this approach, the following code calculates average person location estimates within rating scale categories for the action and feeling items. To find these values, we calculated participants' average rating within each of the item groups rounded to the nearest rating scale category, and then examined the average participant location estimate (θ) from the item-explanatory model within each category.

```
# Item-Explanatory Category Ordering Analyses
## Average person location estimates within categories for
item classifications
### Save person location estimates in a data frame:
lltm_thetas <- unlist(lltm_pcm$persons$id)
lltm_person.locations <- cbind.data.frame(cesd$id, lltm_
thetas)
```

```
names(lltm_person.locations) <- c("id", "theta")
### Set up matrix for results:
n.thresholds <- 3
n.item.groups <- 2
cesd.responses <- subset(cesd, select = -c(id, gender,
living, education))
lltm_category_thetas <- matrix(data = NA, nrow =
n.item.groups, ncol = n.thresholds + 1)
### Use a for-loop to add the results to the matrix:
item.classifications <- c("A", "F", "A", "A", "F", "A", "A",
"A", "A", "A", "F", "A", "F", "A",
"A", "A", "F", "F", "F", "F")
for(item.group in unique(item.classifications)){
group.items <- cbind.data.frame(cesd.responses[,
item.classifications == item.group])
group.item.average <- round(rowMeans(group.items))
group.item.resp <- cbind.data.frame(cesd$id,
group.item.average)
names(group.item.resp) <- c("id", "resp")
cat.0 <- subset(group.item.resp, group.item.resp$resp == 0)
cat.1 <- subset(group.item.resp, group.item.resp$resp == 1)
cat.2 <- subset(group.item.resp, group.item.resp$resp == 2)
cat.3 <- subset(group.item.resp, group.item.resp$resp == 3)
item.group.number <- which(unique(item.classifications) ==
item.group)
merged.cat.0 <- merge(cat.0, lltm_person.locations, by =
"id")
lltm_category_thetas[item.group.number, 1] <-
mean(merged.cat.0$theta)
merged.cat.1 <- merge(cat.1, lltm_person.locations, by =
"id")
lltm_category_thetas[item.group.number, 2] <-
mean(merged.cat.1$theta)
merged.cat.2 <- merge(cat.2, lltm_person.locations, by =
"id")
lltm_category_thetas[item.group.number, 3] <-
mean(merged.cat.2$theta)
merged.cat.3 <- merge(cat.3, lltm_person.locations, by =
"id")
lltm_category_thetas[item.group.number, 4] <-
mean(merged.cat.3$theta)
}
### Label the results:
item.group.category_thetas <- cbind.data.frame(unique
(item.classifications), lltm_category_thetas)
names(item.group.category_thetas) <- c("item_
classification", "x = 0", "x = 1", "x = 2", "x = 3")
### View the results:
View(item.group.category_thetas)
```

Table 8.6 shows the resulting average examinee location estimates from the item-explanatory LLRM within each of the CESD rating scale categories specific to

Table 8.6 Average person location estimates within rating scale categories

Item classification	x=0	x=1	x=2	x=3
Actions	-0.27	0.03	0.42	0.86
Feelings	-0.23	0.06	0.39	0.82

Table 8.7 Rating scale threshold estimates for item classifications

Item classification	τ_1	τ_2	τ_3
Actions	0.55	0.53	1.10
Feelings	0.68	0.31	0.89

the action and feeling item classifications. The increasing average person measures across increasing categories provide support for interpreting the CESD rating scale categories in the intended order for both item classifications.

Next, we will examine threshold parameter estimates as an indicator of category ordering related to the item classifications. Table 8.7 shows the threshold parameter estimates related to the feelings and actions items. These results indicate some ordering concerns related to the first and second threshold for both item types. For the actions items, the first threshold and second threshold are essentially equivalent ($\tau_1 = 0.55$, $\tau_2 = 0.53$); this result suggests the lower rating scale categories may not have been effective for identifying meaningful differences in depression levels for these items. For the feelings items, the second threshold location was notably lower ($\tau_2 = 0.31$) than the first threshold location ($\tau_1 = 0.68$). Together, these results highlight differences in category use between the two item types in the CESD.

Category Precision

To evaluate category precision for the item-explanatory model, we can examine the distance between adjacent pairs of threshold parameters specific to each item classification. In our category ordering analysis, we already observed a negligible difference (0.02 logits) between the first two threshold locations for the actions items. This result suggests that the lower categories in the CESD rating scale may not provide unique insight into participant depression levels as expressed through the actions items. Although the distance between the second and third threshold was larger (0.57 logits), it is still relatively small. Similarly, for the feelings items, the distances were relatively small between both the first and second threshold estimates (0.37 logits) and the second and third threshold estimates (0.58 logits). Together, these results suggest that the four-category CESD rating scale categories may not consistently reflect unique levels of depression for either item classification.

Category Comparability

Our analysis with the item-explanatory model allowed us to check for comparable rating scale functioning between item classifications. As a result, the indicators of category ordering and category precision provided insight into the comparability of category functioning between these item types. Altogether, our results suggested that there are some differences in category functioning between item classifications for the CESD scale.

Rating Scale Analysis with Person-Explanatory Rasch Models

Rating scale analysis with person-explanatory Rasch models involves examining rating scale functioning as it relates to person covariates, such as person subgroups. In this section, we consider this approach using ordinal person subgroups. Specifically, we will use person classifications within education groups in the CESD data to examine differences in rating scale functioning related to person covariates. Using education level as a person-covariate, we can describe our model as a polytomous version of a person-explanatory latent regression Rasch model.

Participants included in our illustrative CESD data reported six education levels, defined as follows: 1 = *eighth grade or less*; 2 = *some high school*; 3 = *completed high school or equivalent*; 4 = *some college or two-year degree*; 5 = *completed four-year college degree*; 6 = *completed graduate or professional degree.* Before running the person-explanatory model using the EIRM package, it is first necessary to ensure that the person classification variable is stored as a factor type. We created a factor version of the education variable in the long-format recoded CESD dataset using the following code.

```
# Change person classifications to factor type:
cesd_long_poly$education.f      <-      as.factor(cesd_long_
poly$education)
```

Next, we specified the equation for the person-explanatory model using the following code:

```
Run the person-explanatory model using education groups:
education_pcm <- eirm(formula = "polyresponse ~ -1 + educa-
tion.f + education.f:polycategory + (1|id)", data = cesd_
long_poly)
```

Our equation includes an interaction between person classifications ("education.f") and the rating scale thresholds ("polycategory"). This specification results in rating scale category threshold estimates that are specific to each education group, which facilitate category comparability analyses. We can extract these results from the model and store them in a matrix using the following code. We will use these threshold values in our rating scale analysis.

```
# Extract threshold parameters:
## Create a matrix with person-classification-specific
threshold difficulty estimates:
n.person.groups <- 6
n.thresholds <- 3
education_pcm.pars <- matrix(data = NA, nrow =
n.person.groups, ncol = n.thresholds)
for(threshold.number in 1:n.thresholds){
if(threshold.number == 1){
education_pcm.pars[, threshold.number] <- -1*education_
pcm$parameters[1:n.person.groups, "Easiness"]
}
if(threshold.number > 1){
education_pcm.pars[, threshold.number] <- -1*education_
pcm$parameters[1:n.person.groups, "Easiness"]-education_
pcm$parameters[(n.person.groups * (threshold.number - 1) +
1):(n.person.groups * threshold.number), "Easiness"]
}
}
View(education_pcm.pars)
```

Rating Scale Category Ordering

We can evaluate rating scale category ordering within each of the education groups using similar methods to those demonstrated earlier with the descriptive PCM and the item-explanatory model. Reflecting this approach, the following code calculates average person location estimates within rating scale categories for each education group. To find these values within each education group, we calculated participants' average rating rounded to the nearest rating scale category, and then examined the average participant location estimate (θ) from the person-explanatory model within each category.

```
# Save person location estimates in a data frame:
education_thetas <- unlist(education_pcm$persons$id)
```

```
education_person.locations <- cbind.data.frame(cesd$id,
education_thetas)
names(education_person.locations) <- c("id", "theta")
# Calculate average person location estimates within cate-
gories for item classifications
## Set up matrix for results:
n.thresholds <- 3
n.item.groups <- 2
cesd.responses <- subset(cesd, select = -c(id, gender,
living, education))
education_category_thetas <- matrix(data = NA, nrow =
n.person.groups, ncol = n.thresholds + 1)
### Use a for-loop to add the results to the matrix:
person.classifications <- cesd$education
for(person.group in c(1:n.person.groups)){
group.items <- cbind.data.frame(cesd.responses
[person.classifications == person.group, ])
group.person.average <- round(rowMeans(group.items))
group.person.resp <- cbind.data.frame(rownames(group.items),
group.person.average)
names(group.person.resp) <- c("id", "resp")
cat.0 <- subset(group.person.resp, group.person.resp$resp =
= 0)
cat.1 <- subset(group.person.resp, group.person.resp$resp =
= 1)
cat.2 <- subset(group.person.resp, group.person.resp$resp =
= 2)
cat.3 <- subset(group.person.resp, group.person.resp$resp =
= 3)
merged.cat.0 <- merge(cat.0, education_person.locations, by
= "id")
education_category_thetas[person.group, 1] <-
mean(merged.cat.0$theta, na.rm = TRUE)
merged.cat.1 <- merge(cat.1, education_person.locations, by
= "id")
education_category_thetas[person.group, 2] <-
mean(merged.cat.1$theta, na.rm = TRUE)
merged.cat.2 <- merge(cat.2, education_person.locations, by
= "id")
education_category_thetas[person.group, 3] <-
mean(merged.cat.2$theta, na.rm = TRUE)
merged.cat.3 <- merge(cat.3, education_person.locations, by
= "id")
education_category_thetas[person.group, 4] <-
mean(merged.cat.3$theta, na.rm = TRUE)
}
### Label the results:
education.group.category_thetas <- cbind.data.frame
(unique(person.classifications), education_category_
thetas)
```

```
names(education.group.category_thetas) <- c("education_
classification", "x = 0", "x = 1", "x = 2", "x = 3")
### View the results:
View(education.group.category_thetas)
```

Table 8.8 shows the resulting average examinee location estimates from the person-explanatory LLRM within each of the CESD rating scale categories specific to the six education groups. Missing values in some cells indicate that, for a given education level, no participants had average ratings within the rating scale category. For example, participants with the lowest education level (eighth grade or less) had average ratings in category 0 on all items. Among the other groups, we observed increasing average person measures across increasing observed categories. These results provide support for interpreting the CESD rating scale categories in the intended order for participants within each of the education level groups, although we note the limited distinction between items for the group with the lowest education level.

Next, we will examine threshold parameter estimates as an indicator of category ordering related to the education groups. Table 8.9 shows the threshold parameter estimates related to the education groups. Consistent with our previous findings, these results indicate some ordering concerns related to the first and second threshold for all participant groups, where the second threshold location is consistently lower than the first threshold location. For participants with education in level 3 (completed

Table 8.8 Average person location estimates within rating scale categories for education level groups

Education group	x=0	x=1	x=2	x=3
1 = Eighth grade or less	0.01	NA	NA	NA
2 = Some high school	-0.32	-0.02	0.38	NA
3 = Completed high school or equivalent	-0.31	0.03	0.42	0.81
4 = Some college or two-year degree	-0.26	0.03	0.44	NA
5 = Completed four-year college degree	-0.28	0.03	0.41	0.88
6 = Completed graduate or professional degree	-0.34	-0.01	0.36	NA

Table 8.9 Rating scale threshold estimates for item classifications

Education Group	τ_1	τ_2	τ_3
1=Eighth grade or less	2.21	1.49	2.18
2=Some high school	0.62	0.09	0.94
3=Completed high school or equivalent	0.53	0.44	1.01
4=Some college or two-year degree	0.59	0.42	0.98
5=Completed four-year college degree	0.50	0.45	1.10
6=Completed graduate or professional degree	0.40	0.37	1.05

high school or equivalent) or higher, the first and second thresholds have nearly equivalent locations. For groups with lower education levels, disordering between these thresholds was more pronounced. However, the second and third thresholds are ordered as expected for all groups.

Category Precision

To evaluate category precision for the person-explanatory model, we can examine the distance between pairs of adjacent threshold parameters specific to each education group. In our category ordering analysis, we observed negligible differences between the first two threshold location estimates for participants in education group 3 (completed high school or equivalent) or higher. This result suggests that the lower categories in the CESD rating scale may not provide unique insight into participant depression levels for participants with relatively higher levels of education. The distance between the second and third thresholds was larger for all groups—indicating more meaningful differences in depression levels reflected in the higher scale categories for all education levels. Together, these results suggest that the four-category CESD rating scale categories may not consistently reflect unique levels of depression.

Category Comparability

Our analysis with the person-explanatory model allowed us to check for comparable rating scale functioning between person subgroups. The indicators of category ordering and category precision within each subgroup provided insight into the comparability of category functioning between groups. Altogether, our results suggested that there are some differences in category functioning between education level subgroups for the CESD scale.

Discussion and Summary

This chapter focused on rating scale analysis, which includes methods for evaluating the degree to which ordinal rating scales function in intended and expected ways. We considered how methods for examining rating scale functioning for descriptive Rasch models, such as the PCM, can be used in a GLMM context, including with explanatory Rasch models. We used an illustrative dataset based on the CESD scale (Radloff, 1977) to demonstrate rating scale analysis with the descriptive PCM and two explanatory Rasch models. Our analyses highlighted differences in rating scale functioning between individual items, item classifications, and between groups of participants. Differences in rating scale functioning identified through such analyses can alert researchers and practitioners to areas where revisions to response scales may be needed and inform the interpretation of responses between items, groups of items, or groups of persons.

Overall, the methods illustrated in this chapter reflect an important aspect of Rasch analyses of polytomous item response data that has practical implications for the interpretation and use of measurement instruments with ordinal response scales. We view rating scale analysis as an essential step in evaluating such instruments that should be included alongside model-data fit analysis. The current chapter connects established rating scale analysis techniques from descriptive Rasch models (e.g., Linacre, 2002; Wind, 2023) to the GLMM framework using explanatory Rasch models.

This chapter has focused on evaluating rating scales. The evaluation of rating scale functioning is closely related to the other topics covered in this book. The combination of item and person covariates in the analyses of rating scales is a rich area for exploration in future research on invariant scales.

References

Adams, R. J., Wu, M. L., & Wilson, M. (2012). The Rasch Rating Model and the Disordered Threshold Controversy. *Educational and Psychological Measurement, 72*(4), 547–573. https://doi.org/10.1177/0013164411432166

Andrich, D. (2011). Rating scales and Rasch measurement. *Expert Review of Pharmacoeconomics & Outcomes Research, 11*, 571–585.

Andrich, D. A. (2013). An Expanded Derivation of the Threshold Structure of the Polytomous Rasch Model That Dispels Any Threshold Disorder Controversy. *Educational and Psychological Measurement, 73*(1), 78–124. https://doi.org/10.1177/0013164412450877

Andrich, D. A. (2015). The problem with the step metaphor for polytomous models for ordinal assessments. *Educational Measurement: Issues and Practice, 34*(2), 8–14. https://doi.org/10.1111/emip.12074

Bulut, O. (2021). *eirm: Explanatory item response modeling for dichotomous and polytomous item responses* (Version 0.3.0) [R]. https://CRAN.R-project.org/package=eirm.

Bulut, O., Gorgun, G., & Yildirim-Erbasli, S. N. (2021). Estimating Explanatory Extensions of Dichotomous and Polytomous Rasch Models: The eirm Package in R. *Psych, 3*(3), Article 3. doi:https://doi.org/10.3390/psych3030023

Engelhard Jr, G., & Wang, J. (2020). *Rasch Models for Solving Measurement Problems* (Vol. 187). Sage. https://us.sagepub.com/en-us/nam/rasch-models-for-solving-measurement-problems/book267292

Fox, J. (2016). *Applied regression analysis and generalized linear models* (Third edition). Sage.

Linacre, J. M. (2002). Optimizing rating scale category effectiveness. *Journal of Applied Measurement, 3*(1), 85–106.

Masters, G. N. (2018). Partial credit model. In W. J. van der Linden (Ed.), *Handbook of Item Response Theory* (Vol. 1, pp. 109–126). CRC Press.

Mellenbergh, G. J. (1995). Conceptual Notes on Models for Discrete Polytomous Item Responses. *Applied Psychological Measurement, 19*(1), 91–100. https://doi.org/10.1177/014662169501900110

Robitzsch, A., Kiefer, T., & Wu, M. (2020). *TAM: Test Analysis Modules* (Version 3.5-19) [Computer software]. https://CRAN.R-project.org/package=TAM

Wetzel, E., & Carstensen, C. H. (2014). Reversed Thresholds in Partial Credit Models: A Reason for Collapsing Categories? *Assessment, 21*(6), 765–774. https://doi.org/10.1177/1073191114530775

Wind, S. A. (2022). Detecting Rating Scale Malfunctioning With the Partial Credit Model and Generalized Partial Credit Model. *Educational and Psychological Measurement, 00131644221116292*. https://doi.org/10.1177/00131644221116292

Wind, S. A. (2023). *Exploring Rating Scale Functioning for Survey Research* (Vol. 193). Sage. https://us.sagepub.com/en-us/nam/exploring-rating-scale-functioning-for-survey-research/book278616

Wright, B. D., & Masters, G. N. (1982). *Rating Scale Analysis: Rasch Measurement*. MESA Press.

Chapter 9
Conclusion

> My focus on invariance is motivated by the claim that we—ordinary people and scientists alike—value invariant relationships … and that they are justified in doing so
>
> (Woodward, 2021, p. 227)

The purpose of this book is to introduce extensions to Rasch models that include the addition of both item and person covariates. The basic family of Rasch models (Wright & Masters, 1984) reflects descriptive measurement models. This book describes explanatory item response models within the framework of Rasch measurement theory that can be used to explore and predict item response probabilities using item and person variables (covariates) that can be explicitly included in the measurement model. Item covariates can be used to provide additional validity evidence by exploring variables that predict item locations on the latent variable using item characteristics, such as content and cognitive demand. Likewise, person covariates also add to our understanding of the meaning of the responses and scores by examining how the items function for individuals and subgroups within the larger pool of people for whom the scale is designed to be used.

The analyses described in this book offer methodological tools that can be used to delve more deeply into person responses to a set of items designed to represent a latent variable or construct. It is important to note that there are lots of choices to estimate different explanatory item response models—as always, the models selected should be guided by the research questions and the purpose of the study. The substantive interpretation of these models requires careful attention to the underlying form of the model.

Each of these chapters adds to an overall perspective on the next generation of invariant measurement. We consider each chapter in turn with the goal of highlighting the implications of each chapter for the next generation of invariant measurement. Figure 9.1, as originally shown in the preface reflects an overview of all of the chapters.

G. Engelhard and S. A. Wind, *Invariant Measurement with Explanatory Rasch Models in the Human Sciences*, https://doi.org/10.1007/978-3-032-08816-1_9

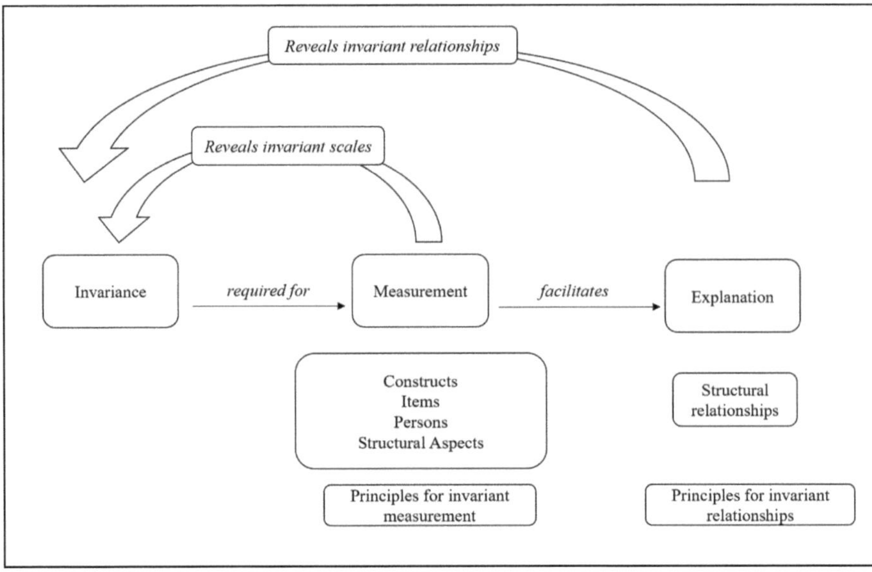

Fig. 9.1 Principles for invariance

Summary and Implications of Each Chapter

The first chapter provided a general introduction to the themes of the book. Chapter 1 described the essential principles of Rasch measurement theory with an introduction to the Dichotomous Model using an application with the Learning Stimulation Scale for measuring home environments. The Dichotomous Model is the most basic descriptive Rasch model that includes the essential features of invariant measurement. Chapter 1 also introduced the concept of explanatory Rasch models. Explanatory Rasch models are at the core of this book with an emphasis on extending the basic features of invariant measurement to consider invariant relationships between stable measures. Each of the descriptive Rasch models can be modified to become explanatory models by including item and person covariates. These covariates can be used to collect additional evidence regarding the potential meaning and use of the scores, and determine conditions in which invariant measurement may not be achieved. Explanatory models seek to provide evidence regarding why relationships are invariant, and the conditions that may limit this invariance. As pointed out by Wright, "science is impossible without an evolving network of stable measures" (p. 33). These networks reflect the inter-relationships between latent variables identified in our theories of human behavior.

Chapters 2 and 3 presented the foundations of Rasch measurement theory, which is the "glue" that holds the entire volume together. Chapter 2 developed the historical and philosophical principles of Rasch measurement theory, while Chap. 3 introduced the use of generalized linear mixed models (GLMMs) to estimate the parameters of various extensions to descriptive Rasch models that can be used for explanatory purposes.

Chapter 2 introduced the basic historical and philosophical underpinnings of measurement, explanation, and invariance. We discussed how most measurement models can be considered descriptive in nature. Then, we introduced the idea that explanation can and should be included within measurement broadly conceived. Chapter 2 began with a discussion of invariance including a historical overview of how key measurement theorists (Guttman, Lazarsfeld, Mokken, and Rasch) approached invariance within the context of measurement. Next, we extended the concept of invariance to explanation by considering path analysis, factor analysis, structural equation models, and explanatory models. These extensions reflect aspects of science, and its connections to invariance with regards to relationships between latent variables. We discussed the combination of Rasch principles related to measurement, explanation, and invariance. This chapter emphasized that an important goal of measurement is to create scales that yield meaningful and useful scores that are "stable when our backs turned." We introduced the idea that next generation of invariant measurement research should include both description and explanation in measurement models. Invariance is a hallmark of measurement and explanation. Discovering the conditions under which measures and relationships are invariant includes directly considering and exploring the factors that place limits on this invariance.

Chapter 3 focused on estimating the Dichotomous Model using GLMMs. We provided a brief review and summary of linear models, mixed models, generalized linear models, and generalized linear mixed models. We presented an underlying statistical framework of generalized linear mixed models for estimating the parameters of the Dichotomous Model. We used the Learning Stimulation Scale to illustrate this approach with analyses performed using the EIRM package in R (Bulut, 2021).

Evaluation of measurement quality in Rasch measurement theory is based on model-data fit, and this issue is addressed in Chap. 4. We continued our analysis of the Learning Stimulation Scale with a focus on model-data fit. Rasch measurement theory describes the requirements that must be approximated with real data in order to achieve the twin goals of person-invariant item calibration and item-invariant measurement of persons. We described how Rasch's approach is fundamentally different from other measurement and statistical approaches to data analyses. Standard statistical models focus on obtaining the best fit to observed data with the model modified to obtain better model-data fit. In Rasch measurement theory, we start with a strong theory of measurement, and then proactively examine data to test for invariant measurement. A key part of these model-data fit analyses is the diagnostic value of identifying misfitting items and persons. For example, a person with an unusual response pattern may not have engaged in a meaningful way with the items due to other factors, such as boredom or guessing. Item misfit may happen when an item includes a confusing stem or unclear response options on a selected-response item. In order to evaluate measurement quality, model-data fit analysis is organized around various statistical and graphical analyses of residuals. Residuals reflect the difference between observed responses and model-based expected responses. It is important to recognize that the invariance properties of Rasch measurement theory are only achieved when good model-data fit is obtained.

Chapter 5 went in depth into the use of generalized linear mixed models for estimating explanatory Rasch models. This chapter provided specific details for two models: the Linear Logistic Rasch Model (LLRM) and the latent regression Rasch model (LRRM). We used the Learning Stimulation Scale and the Attitude Toward Censorship (ATC) Scale to illustrate both models. We used the LLRM to analyze the Learning Stimulation Scale with an item covariate classifying the items as child or adult activities. Then, we used the LRRM to analyze the ATC Scale with both an item covariate and two person covariates. For the ATC Scale, valence (sentiment implied by the words in the stem of the item: negative, neutral, positive) was included as an item covariate in the Linear Logistic Rasch Model, while two person covariates (education level and gender) were included in latent regression Rasch model. A detailed description of how to analyze the ATC Scale was provided, including the substantive interpretation of the parameters of the models. This chapter also described in detail the descriptive and explanatory versions of these models. The analyses included both dichotomous responses (Learning Stimulation Scale) and polytomous responses (ATC Scale).

Chapter 6 explored the use of explanatory Rasch models for analyzing rater-mediated assessments. Rater-mediated assessments are based in a fundamental way on the ratings obtained from raters. Essentially, raters engage in a judgmental process to score constructed responses or performances using a rating scale that represents a construct. A person's score or rating is mediated through the rater. We used an analysis of data from a high school writing test administered to students in the United States. The analyses were primarily conducted using the TAM package in R (Robitzsch et al., 2020). We used a combination of descriptive Many-Facet Rasch Models (MFRM) and explanatory MRFMs to analyze the data and consider how invariant measurement and explanatory Rasch models apply in the context of rater-mediated assessments.

Chapter 7 described five components for instrument development (construct, observational design, scoring rules, measurement model, and structural aspects) that can be used when a researcher is constructing a scale based on the principles of Rasch measurement theory with an explanatory modeling approach. We discussed and illustrated how explanatory Rasch models can support instrument development for measurement across a variety of contexts. The principles were illustrated with data from a Transitive Reasoning Scale (TRS). We analyzed the TRS data using Explanatory Rasch Models that included an item covariate (number of items) and a person covariate (student grade level). We used the glmer function in R to estimate the models (Bates et al., 2024). Our second illustration was based on data from a biology assessment, and we used the EIRM package (Bulut, 2021) to estimate the models. We included two item covariates (cognitive demand and content). This chapter illustrated some of the ways that explanatory Rasch models can be used to inform the item and test development process. There is a need a more research to explore how these models can be integrated into the ongoing processes within a broader measurement context.

Finally, Chap. 8 provided a compact introduction to rating scale analysis for polytomous explanatory Rasch models. The focus was on methods for evaluating the degree to which ordinal rating scales function in the intended and expected ways based on Rasch measurement theory. We discussed methods for examining rating scale functioning for descriptive Rasch models, such as the Partial Credit Model (PCM) and Rating Scale Model (RSM), within the GLMM context. We extended the descriptive models to include explanatory Rasch models with rating scales. We used the CESD scale to demonstrate rating scale analysis with the descriptive PCM and two explanatory Rasch models. Our analyses highlighted differences in rating scale functioning between individual items, item classifications, and between groups of participants. Differences in rating scale functioning identified through such analyses can alert researchers and practitioners to areas where revisions to response scales may be needed and inform the interpretation of responses between items, groups of items, or groups of persons.

Where Do we Go from Here?

As this book goes to press, there is a great deal of discussion of the role of generative AI in education and measurement (Baek & Wilson, 2024; Hao et al., 2024). Generative AI is essentially a subset of artificial intelligence that focuses on creating new content based on patterns and structures learned from existing data. The goal of generative AI is to create original data that mimics the training data, while traditional AI analyzes data to make predictions and classifications

Recently, Lee and Engelhard (2024) considered some of the features of next generation assessments and the role of Rasch measurement theory. They identified four key features of next generation assessments that are expected to be based on personalized assessments that are technology-based using generative AI within digital environments.

First, next generation assessments will be personalized with a focus on individuals. One feature of personalized assessments is that they can offer the opportunity for contextualized learning by identifying prior knowledge, and then tailoring individual students with different instructional strategies. For example, Yuan et al. (2022)) described an approach for identifying targeted feedback strategies for student writing. It is interesting that this is related to an early observation of Rasch (1960/1980) in the introduction to his book. He pointed out that measurement had been previously criticized for focusing on groups in contrast to the individual-based statistics—Rasch measurement theory provides insight into individual responses that reflect the spirit of personalized assessment.

Next generation assessments will be technology-based. For example, new formats for administering, developing, and scoring tests have been developing at lightning speed (ITC-ATP, 2022). Each of these formats pose new psychometric challenges, and Rasch measurement theory holds promise for evaluating the psychometric quality of these technological innovations, and their impact on assessment systems.

Thirdly, generative AI undergirds many aspects of assessment processes. It is important to consider the ethical guidelines for using AI, such as those suggested by UNESCO (2024). The core principles are Proportionality and Do No Harm, Safety and Security, Right to Privacy and Data Protection, Multi-stakeholder and Adaptive Governance & Collaboration, Responsibility and Accountability, Transparency and Explainability, Human Oversight and Determination, Sustainability, Awareness & Literacy, and Fairness and Non-Discrimination. A detailed exploration of these guidelines is beyond the scope of this chapter, but each of these guidelines can be considered in detail within the context of next generation assessments using Rasch measurement theory.

Finally, digital environments will host and support the next generation of assessments. One of the challenges with digital environments is the need for privacy to protect the rights of individual test-takers. Digital environments offer numerous benefits; however, they also present challenges, including ethical concerns and potential misuses. As digital environments evolve and new advances emerge, it is crucial to address limitations and to harness the full potential to improve assessment systems.

In summary, we are confident that invariant measurement and Rasch measurement theory can play an important role as the world considers another new technology (generative AI) with great potential for good, and great potential for harmful unintended consequences.

References

Baek, E. O., & Wilson, R. V. (2024). An inquiry into the use of generative AI and its implications in education: Boon or bane. *International Journal of Adult Education and Technology, 15*(1), 1–14.

Bates, D., Maechler, M., Bolker, B., & Walker, S. (2024). *lme4: Linear Mixed-Effects Models using "Eigen" and S4* (Version 1.1–35.5, p. 1.1–35.5) [R]. https://CRAN.R-project.org/package=lme4

Bulut, O. (2021). *EIRM: Explanatory item response modeling for dichotomous and polytomous item responses* [Computer software]. Retrieved from http://CRAN.R-project.org/package=EIRM.

Hao, J., von Davier, A. A., Yaneva, V., Lottridge, S., von Davier, M., & Harris, D. J. (2024). Transforming assessment: The impacts and implications of large language models and generative AI. *Educational Measurement: Issues and Practice, 43*(2), 16–29.

International Test Commission and Association of Test Publishers. (2022). *Guidelines for technology-based assessment*. Association of Test Publishers.

Lee, E., & Engelhard, G. (2024). Next generation assessments and Rasch measurement theory. *Rasch Measurement Transactions, 37*, 1956–1959.

Masters, G. N., & Wright, B. D. (1984). The essential process in a family of measurement models. *Psychometrika, 49*, 529–544.

Robitzsch, A., Kiefer, T., & Wu, M. (2020). *TAM: Test Analysis Modules* (3.5–19) [Computer software]. https://CRAN.R-project.org/package=TAM

UNESCO. (2024). Ethics of artificial intelligence. Retrieved November 06, 2024, from https://www.unesco.org/en/artificialintelligence/recommendation-ethics

Yuan, Y., Engelhard, G., Jr., Raczynski, K., & Wang, J. (2022). Using unfolding models to identify targeted feedback strategies for student writing. *Assessing Writing, 54*.

Index

A
Attitude Toward Censorship (ATC), 93, 99–102, 104–110, 216

B
Biology Exam, 175–182, 184

C
Category Functioning, 205, 209
Category Probability Curves, 144, 147, 197, 198
Center for Epidemiological Studies Depression (CESD), 188–191, 193–201, 203–205, 208, 209, 217
Construct Validity, 72
Covariates, 1, 5, 11, 36, 37, 39, 42, 43, 57, 59, 65, 75, 85, 93, 95–99, 106, 109, 110, 116, 117, 159, 161–163, 166, 171, 173, 176–178, 180, 184, 200, 201, 213, 214, 216

D
Dichotomous Rasch Model, 49, 56, 59, 60, 64, 66, 71, 77, 78, 85, 89, 91, 163, 165, 167–170, 176, 177, 179, 180, 182, 184
Differential Item Functioning, 20, 34, 42, 43

E
Explanatory Rasch Models, 1–3, 8, 12, 15, 32, 35, 38, 39, 43, 45, 56, 70, 72, 75, 82, 91, 93, 95, 96, 99, 106, 108, 110, 114–116, 125–128, 133, 136, 138, 149, 151–153, 157, 167, 171, 176, 177, 180, 184, 185, 187, 188, 190, 193, 200, 201, 205, 209, 210, 214, 216, 217

F
Fair Average, 139
Fixed Effects, 11, 36, 37, 54, 56, 59, 95, 96, 167, 171, 174, 175

G
Generalized Linear Mixed Models (GLMM), 1, 8, 11, 12, 20, 36, 49, 54, 56–58, 60, 93, 95, 96, 98, 106, 109, 110, 171, 190, 191, 209, 210, 214–217
Generative AI, 217, 218

I
Infit, 65, 66, 72, 73, 76, 84, 85, 88, 90, 91, 133, 134, 136–138, 142
Instrument Development, 157–163, 176, 177, 184, 216
Invariant Measurement, 1, 2, 4, 5, 12, 28, 32, 39, 40, 44, 45, 63, 64, 89, 114, 115, 152, 153, 213–216, 218
Item Fit Statistics, 76, 84
Item-Invariant, 2, 4, 17, 39, 40, 215

G. Engelhard and S. A. Wind, *Invariant Measurement with Explanatory Rasch Models in the Human Sciences*, https://doi.org/10.1007/978-3-032-08816-1

L

Latent Regression Rasch Model (LRRM), 11, 37, 42, 77, 93, 103, 106, 107, 110, 165, 205, 216
Learning Stimulation Scale, 8–11, 49, 55, 57, 58, 60, 64, 73, 77–79, 81, 83–86, 88–90, 93, 96–99, 110, 214–216
Linear Logistic Rasch Model (LLRM), 11, 37, 42, 65, 75, 93, 95–99, 104, 106, 110, 163, 165, 170–174, 176, 177, 180, 183, 201, 203, 208, 216
Link Function, 37, 54, 56, 95
Local Independence, 21–23, 26, 27, 65, 67–69, 80

M

Many-Facet Rasch Model (MFRM), 93, 115–120, 122–128, 132–134, 136, 139, 142, 143, 148, 152, 153, 216
Measurement Invariance, 20, 33, 34, 42, 43
Measurement Model, 1, 11, 12, 16, 20, 31, 34, 36, 40–43, 45, 76, 96, 110, 125, 158, 161, 162, 165, 176, 177, 180, 184, 195, 199, 213, 215, 216
Measurement Quality, 63, 64, 71, 89, 91, 126, 161, 215
Model-data fit, 27, 33, 36, 45, 58, 60, 63–65, 67–72, 74–79, 82, 84, 85, 89, 91, 103, 104, 107, 119, 120, 125, 128, 131, 133, 134, 136, 137, 139, 142, 161, 210, 215, 216

O

Observational Design, 160, 163, 176, 178, 184, 216
Outfit, 65, 66, 72, 73, 76, 84, 85, 88–91, 133, 134, 136–138, 142

P

Partial Credit Model, 11, 93, 95, 98, 99, 103, 104, 107, 116, 187, 188, 217
Personalized Assessments, 217
Person Covariates, 1, 20, 36, 42, 43, 45, 66, 70, 71, 77, 85, 93, 95, 99, 103, 106, 109, 110, 117, 159, 163, 176, 200, 201, 205, 210, 213, 214, 216

R

Random Effects, 11, 36, 37, 54, 56, 57, 59, 83, 96, 167, 171, 174
Rater Errors, 114, 125, 137, 138, 153
Rater-Mediated, 60, 113–116, 120, 122–129, 131–133, 136, 137, 142, 143, 149, 151–153, 216
Rater Severity, 116, 118, 119, 123, 125, 127, 129, 131, 136, 139, 141, 149, 150, 152, 153
Rating Scale Model, 11, 93, 95, 98, 99, 104–107, 217
Residual Analysis/ Residual Analyses, 64, 67, 73, 86

S

Scoring Designs, 125–128, 153
Scoring Rules, 159–161, 163, 165, 177, 178, 184, 216
Separation Reliability, 65, 66, 74, 77, 85, 86, 88, 89, 118, 128–131, 133, 137
Specific Objectivity, 3, 12, 20, 28–30, 40, 41, 71, 89
Structural Aspects, 34, 40–43, 65, 66, 71, 75, 77, 95, 157–159, 161–163, 165, 176, 177, 180, 184, 216

T

Threshold Parameters, 98, 120, 121, 143, 187, 192, 199, 200, 202, 204, 208, 209
Thresholds, 120, 129, 130, 133, 148, 190, 192, 193, 195, 196, 199–201, 206, 209
Transitive Reasoning, 157, 162, 163, 165–174, 176, 180, 184

U

Unidimensional Scale, 2, 18, 20, 26, 40, 67

V

Validity Evidence, 97, 213

W

Wright Map, 2, 57, 59–61, 64, 66, 86, 89, 115, 128, 131–133, 142, 143, 169, 170, 173, 174, 179, 180

MIX
Papier aus verantwortungsvollen Quellen
Paper from responsible sources
FSC® C105338

If you have any concerns about our products,
you can contact us on
ProductSafety@springernature.com

In case Publisher is established outside the EU,
the EU authorized representative is:
Springer Nature Customer Service Center GmbH
Europaplatz 3, 69115 Heidelberg, Germany

Printed by Libri Plureos GmbH
in Hamburg, Germany